SACRED BLISS

SACRED BLISS

A Spiritual History
of **CANNABIS**

MARK S. FERRARA

ROWMAN & LITTLEFIELD
Lanham • Boulder • New York • London

Published by Rowman & Littlefield
A wholly owned subsidiary of
The Rowman & Littlefield Publishing Group, Inc.
4501 Forbes Boulevard, Suite 200, Lanham, Maryland 20706
https://rowman.com

Unit A, Whitacre Mews, 26-34 Stannary Street, London SE11 4AB,
United Kingdom

British Library Cataloguing in Publication Information Available

Library of Congress Cataloging-in-Publication Data
Names: Ferrara, Mark S., author.
Title: Sacred bliss : a spiritual history of Cannabis / Mark S. Ferrara.
Description: Lanham : Rowman & Littlefield Publishing Group, Inc., [2016] |
    Includes bibliographical references and index.
Identifiers: LCCN 2016022787 (print) | LCCN 2016031856 (ebook) | ISBN
    9781442271913 (hardcover : alk. paper) | ISBN 9781442271920 (electronic)
Subjects: LCSH: Hallucinogenic drugs and religious experience. | Cannabis. |
    Marijuana.
Classification: LCC BL65.D7 F47 2016 (print) | LCC BL65.D7 (ebook) | DDC
    204/.2—dc23
LC record available at http://lccn.loc.gov/2016022787

∞ ™ The paper used in this publication meets the minimum requirements of
American National Standard for Information Sciences Permanence of Paper for
Printed Library Materials, ANSI/NISO Z39.48-1992.

Printed in the United States of America

For Walter Raleigh Coppedge—erudite adventurer, determined educator, and steadfast friend—whose "Yes!" to life inspires all who know him

CONTENTS

ACKNOWLEDGMENTS

No book-length project of this nature comes together without a fortunate alignment of circumstances; such a happy confluence of events led me to the University of California at Berkeley during the spring of 2015 as a visiting scholar in the English Department. Access to the extensive collections in the University of California at Berkeley libraries made the timely completion of the first draft of *Sacred Bliss: A Spiritual History of Cannabis* possible.

My wife, Liangmei Bao, lent her support to yet another book project, this time braving several weeks of a snowy winter in upstate New York alone—while I wrote (guiltily) in California. Howbeit, one is hard-pressed to find a better place to write a book on cannabis culture given the importance of the San Francisco Bay area as a site for the religious and scientific exploration of consciousness from the 1950s to 1970s, the role of the University of California's flagship campus in protecting free speech and promoting tolerance of a diversity of expression, and the state's establishment of the first medical marijuana program in the nation in 1996.

I am honor-bound to acknowledge ample parental support along with the generous guidance of several former professors, most notably Walter Coppedge (to whom this study is dedicated), Cliff Edwards, Marcel Cornis-Pope, and W. Scott Howard. Many thanks are due also to the kind folks who reviewed sections of the manuscript, including J. Jeremy Wisnewski, Wesley Graves, Arnaud Brichon, Sabine Assad, Geoffrey and Shirley O'Shea, Bryan Walpert, Toke Knudsen, Brian Dolber, Michael

Rinella, Wendy Lochner, Hope Von Stengel, R. A. Brown, Dan Alexander, and Nicole Ann Jones. Of course, the claims herein—and errors of fact—are mine alone.

Whenever possible, I wrote on the patio of the La Posada Guest House near campus. There the amiable trio of Irma Reyna, Ada Ormsby, and Vilma Hernandez safeguarded a quiet place for me under the shade of a canvas gazebo. In their lovely little garden, the exuberance of nature was on full display in a proliferation of flowers, in the fluttering of humming-bird wings, in the mischievous antics of blue jays, and in the caws of shiny crows waiting to clean one's bones—a strong incentive to work!

On the road trips from New York to California, and back, Liangmei and I met friends and family along the way, including the gifted painter and musician Michael Peter Robinson (son of artist Ione Robinson) in New Mexico; Qiao and her husband Bryce in Utah; Busdriver, Rainbow Mountain, and Vinnie in Colorado; Charlie Nelson, Tim Knepper, Kirk Martin, Pat Bell, and Dina Smith in Iowa; Matt Voorhees and Kristy King in Arizona; and Jim and Cory Ferrara (and kin) in California.

The visit to Berkeley also made possible conversations with some remarkable people, such as the physician and early advocate for cannabis medicine Frank H. Lucido, poet and novelist Kathleen Spivack (daughter of economist Peter Drucker), composer and writer Debora Simcovich, the ever-cheerful and thoughtful Thomas Holenstein of ETH Zürich, Nancy and Jennifer Cooke, Thomas Reardon and Sasha Volberg at Michigan State University, George Bertelstein at the Medicine Path Native American Church in Berkeley, and bandleader Eric Van James.

Harborside Health Center in Oakland merits commendation for bringing cannabis medicine "out of the shadows, into the light," as does the nation's longest continuously operating dispensary, Berkeley Patients Group, for pioneering those efforts. A United University Professions Individual Development Award, and professional development funding from the Department of English at SUNY Oneonta, helped to offset some of the expenditures associated with researching and writing this volume. I thank the student-staff at the University of California at Berkeley libraries (who pulled hundreds of books for me); their bright intelligence and cheerful diligence fills one with hope.

INTRODUCTION

Cannabis, Consciousness, and Healing

A revolutionary experiment is underway in the United States. At the time of writing, twenty-three states and the District of Columbia have enacted laws permitting the use of marijuana medicine. Alaska, Washington, Colorado, and Oregon have legalized cannabis altogether and now seek to create commercial regulatory systems for its production, distribution, and taxation. Arizona, California, Massachusetts, Maine, Nevada, and other states will likely follow that lead in the 2016 election cycle.

The net effect of these and other transformations in social attitudes is that more people now enjoy greater access to cannabis, for medical and recreational purposes, than before the enforcement provisions of the 1937 Marihuana Tax Act rendered impossible the handling, dispensing, selling, or giving of it in the United States. For this reason, Americans living in locales with progressive medical and legal statutes—and people around the world like them—have a unique opportunity for engagement with cannabis on a more profound level of mental and physical healing.

This study differs from other book-length investigations of cannabis, for it contains no instructions regarding its cultivation, no scientific discussions of its botany, and no rankings of potent strains. Nor is it a cookbook, a history of the prohibition of marijuana, or a political treatise urging lawmakers to end the practice of incarceration for possession without the intent to distribute. This book does not even describe the primary chemical compounds in cannabis, or explain their effects on human physiology as they are metabolized. Nor will it provide a scientific rationale for the efficacy of marijuana medicine in treating dozens of ailments (from arthritis to multiple sclerosis, asthma to post-traumatic stress disorder).

Scholars and laypersons have fitfully probed these and other topics and their work constitutes a growing body of literature that maps out the history, pharmacology, and growing social import of marijuana in the United States and around the globe. By contrast, *Sacred Bliss* explores the role of cannabis in inducing, augmenting, and sustaining spiritual awakening. To make that venture as meaningful as possible, we engage sacred and secular texts from around the world in which cannabis appears—and *historically and culturally contextualize their core themes.*

In this sense, the book that you have in your hands is a religious history of marijuana with an emphasis on finding *presence* in daily life by way of direct experience. Written for the seeker, not the pedant, *Sacred Bliss* makes the case for cannabis as a mild entheogen, one of many substances that help people to "discover God within" by acting as "universal keys that unlock the door within each of our minds to other forms of consciousness."[1]

The increasing utilization of medical cannabis to alleviate the pain and symptoms of physiological disease raises the possibility of employing current treatment regimes to heal the mind, along with the body. For patients facing terminal diagnoses, who take marijuana as a way to manage the side effects of synthetic medications and treatment regimes, such as chemotherapy, the cultivation of an intensely aware acceptance of the here-now may provide comfort by pointing beyond identification with the physical body and toward an understanding of the universal and enduring nature of the true self.

Many of the medical and religious traditions explored in this book precede Western science in acknowledging the full implications of the relationship between human consciousness and the physical body. The regular meditator on the spiritual path open to the use of a mild entheogen as an aid in focusing attention will find herein a detailed survey of religious traditions that integrate cannabis into the effort to reveal inner divinity, blur the boundary between self and other, and discern the infinite within all material forms as the ego dissolves and new vistas of reality unfurl. From that religious perspective, one recognizes the power of marijuana to help awaken a universal sense of I-am-ness, sacredness, and experience of union.

The following chapters offer recreational consumers, enjoying new freedoms in progressive states such as Colorado and Oregon, alternative ways to engage the creative mental space that cannabis opens, so as to make experiences with it more meaningful and potentially life altering. For the broadminded non-user, this book extends forays into wellness, expanded perception, and holistic healing grounded in an engagement with scripture. Wendy Chapkis and Richard J. Webb note that marijuana ranks among the safest therapeutically active plant substances known to mankind, since it is impossible to ingest enough to induce a lethal response (as a result of drug-related toxicity).[2] This fact makes cannabis safer than many commonly consumed foods, and more important, it offers partakers an augmented sense of wellness, access to higher levels of productivity (contrary to stereotypes), and a calm tolerance accompanying longtime use that may be employed to put the breath and mind in accord.

Of course, the shifts in perception, mood, and memory that broadly characterize the psychoactive properties of marijuana are highly dependent on circumstance and intention. Anyone who has taken cannabis in complex social settings understands that it may evoke feelings of isolation that generate anxiety, whereas in intimate and peaceful environments (perhaps among good friends or in the midst of striking natural beauty) it brings stillness to the fore of consciousness and clarifies perception. For this reason alone, many musicians and artists use cannabis to nuance hearing and seeing before, during, and after the act of creation. Consumed in situations conducive to contemplation, and with right intention, marijuana stimulates introspection and the "stoned realizations" that come with thoughts about mortality, an individual's relationship to God, and the difficulty of awakening (or accessing grace). From that perspective, the medical or recreational use of marijuana does not constitute an escape from reality—rather it may propel one directly toward it.

In anticipation of our discussion of the role of marijuana in the world's religious traditions, we must understand the nature of what Abraham Maslow termed "peak-experiences" (naturally occurring "mystical," "transcendental," "psychedelic," "self-transcendent," or "unitive" experiences). Maslow found that tremendous concentration drives all peak-experiences, and through them, the truest and most total kind of perceiv-

ing takes place. In such a state of consciousness, human cognition becomes "non-evaluating," "noncomparing," and "nonjudging" of its own
volition as it rests quietly in heightened awareness.[3] Peak-experiences
occur in every time, culture, religious tradition, economic class, and gender, and they exemplify a form of religious revelation that has played a
pivotal role in the history of religion.[4]

During peak-experiences, the universe is perceived as an integrated
whole, and that fact is directly discoverable in the "minute particulars"[5]
of the physical world—a flower, a blade of grass, or the bare branches of
a tree against a blue sky. Such clear discernment of the luminous essence
pervading all material forms abides in the experienced practitioner and
culminates in a collapse of the distinction between self and other. In most
of us, however, peak-experiences are infrequent and fleeting occurrences
that offer only glimpses of reality. Yet a single such encounter with the
divine can test otherwise automatic attachment to the preconceptions that
limit perception—that is, the prejudgment which is the literal meaning of
prejudice.

In *Religions, Values, and Peak-Experiences*, Maslow argues that although they contain "ethnocentric phrasings," making them dependent on
time, place, and cultural origin, the ineffable that peak-experiences open
toward is universal and accessible to anyone at any time.[6] Although feelings of wonder, awe, reverence, humility, profound gratitude, and surrender attend peak-experiences, due to their radically subjective nature, like
a finger pointing toward the moon, words cannot present reality; they can
only clumsily re-present it. For this reason, they are often articulated
using negation and paradox: their truth cannot be expressed in words
because the divine is uncreated, undifferentiated, indivisible, unmanifest,
unnamable, formless, the ground of being, and so forth.

When the world is thus perceived as beautiful, good, and desirable, it
results in a greater acceptance of all aspects of life, including those once
rejected as unwelcome (such as ill health) despite their actuality.[7] As
mindfulness of being (or to use Maslow's term, B-cognition) attending
peak-experiences settles in, one becomes more receptive to the way
things are—and thereby all manner of self-perpetuated contradiction and
conflict in life comes to an end. B-cognition is ego transcending, self-
forgetting, utterly unselfish—and that absence of desire or resistance by
the ego is often described symbolically as an act of dying.[8] As Jesus
acknowledges in the Gospel of John, "unless one is born anew, he cannot

see the kingdom of God."[9] We will encounter similar directives multiple times during our journey.

B-cognition also severs automatic identification with the stream of incessant "self-talk" that characterizes everyday consciousness and is often misconstrued as the true self. What Maslow called "unitive consciousness" emerges from glimpses of the sacred (the extraordinary) in the ordinary everyday world.[10] In the usual mode of cognition, by contrast, mental noise makes it difficult to distinguish the real from the unreal—the thing itself from one's thoughts, ideologies, and prejudgments about it. By contrast, B-cognition spurns the fixation on reconstructed pasts and imagined futures that is the usual habit of thought, and in doing so transcends time and space as ordinarily experienced. When the incessant grasping of the mind is thus apprehended and intuitively understood, it ceases of its own accord. Zen master Dōgen Zenji referred to this mode of being as one of "dropped off body and mind."[11]

Such a state of awareness comes with the recognition that one is not the continual stream of thoughts—but the conscious space in which they emerge along with everything else, out of emptiness moment after moment: birds chirping, lawn mowers buzzing, cars zipping by, people talking, thoughts coming and going—"all that jazz." Brief moments of "awakening" interrupt otherwise automatic identification with thought, and direct attention to the unity of the present moment. The experience of the fundamental nonduality of inner and outer (that "all things are one"), which accompanies B-cognition, instills a deep sense of purpose in life, facilitates open-mindedness, and results in lower value being assigned to material gain, dogmatic belief, and social status.

Immediately recognizing their centrality to mental and physical health, Maslow made peak-experiences an important marker of self-actualization, the impulse to realize one's full potential. Readers familiar with his theory of the hierarchy of needs will recall that self-transcendence sits atop a pyramidal structure (supported by a pattern of motivations whereby an individual's physiological, safety, belongingness, and self-esteem needs are met prior to self-actualization). Maslow's psychological account of peak-experiences provides us with a secular and scientific entry point for this historical survey of cannabis in religion, culture, and medicine, for he ascertained that individuals in whom peak-experiences unfolded could be cured of "chronic anxiety and neurosis," "existential meaninglessness," and even "obsessional thoughts of suicide."[12] In such people, the here-now takes on added import, thereby allowing them to live more fully from the creative center of being without fretting, striving, or yearning.[13]

The ingestion of mild psychoactive substances such as marijuana has stimulated peak-experiences since the dawn of human history, and we understand that in their truest form, they are indistinguishable from naturally occurring mystical experiences brought forth by meditation, prayer, or other "religious" activity.[14] The gradual decriminalization and legalization of marijuana now makes possible extended explorations of consciousness using an entheogen whose effects are less dramatic than those of LSD, psilocybin, peyote, or other hard psychedelics. Although the latter substances remain highly regulated in the eyes of the law (if unjustly so), Aldous Huxley, Alan Watts, Richard Alpert (Ram Dass), John Lilly, Timothy Leary, and scores of others have written at length concerning their benefits, dangers, and limitations. In contrast to the abrupt shifts in consciousness ("good trips" and "bad trips") reported by these Western pioneers of twentieth-century psychedelia, the potential for marijuana to more subtly expand perception often goes overlooked, while its shallower physical and mental side effects (such as dryness of the mouth and eyes, stimulation of hunger, and mild spatial and temporal reorientation) become the fodder of late-night comedians.

In low dosages, such as those achieved by inhalation and through tinctures, cannabis produces a mild euphoric effect employed by shamans and herbal healers across time and culture. Higher dosages of cannabis, usually gained by the consumption of potent edibles, produce stronger and longer-lasting effects that may be accompanied by hot or cold flashes, even panic and hallucination in some individuals.[15] Those consuming medical marijuana edibles learn to titrate their dosages to control symptoms for maximum therapeutic effect without these and other relatively rare side effects. With cannabis now legally and effectively treating the symptoms of so many severe illnesses, more attention deserves to be given to its ability to open the doorway to peak-experiences—especially in those facing chronic maladies or the end of life. For some, death is easier to embrace if the illusion of self and other is cut asunder, even if for a short moment.

In the chapters that follow, the attributes of marijuana that have made it a part of medicine, ritual, and spiritual practice since prehistory in Asia, Africa, and the Middle East are underscored. Our exploration of that deployment of cannabis around the globe begins in India during the Vedic period (c. 1700 BCE to 600 CE). In chapter 1, "Vedānta, Sādhu Priests, and the 'Lord of Bhang,'" early Indian religion is interpreted in light of the ancient animism preserved in the *Rig Veda* and the *Atharva Veda* (which designates marijuana as a "sacred grass" and celebrates it as one of five hallowed plants). As it evolved, Hindu philosophy became resolutely nondualistic, and Brahmin priests discovered marijuana in its various forms including hashish and bhang as beneficial to the realization of moksha (awakening or liberation). This holy herb features prominently in contemporary ritual offerings to Lord Shiva, as well.

In chapter 2, "Shamans, Sufis, and the 'Green Man,'" we move from South Asia to Persia and Anatolia in the Middle East, where Iranian Zoroastrian shamans sought to replicate the religious experiences of their tradition's founder by smoking cannabis to induce ecstasy. Prior to the arrival of Islam in the seventh century, the *Avesta* scripture referenced hashish as a beneficial narcotic—and Mithraic sacrifices included the ritualistic consumption of psychoactive plants to alter consciousness and create a space where ritually purified foods could be shared between humans and the divinities. While the *Quran* strictly prohibits intoxicants that "cover" the mind such as alcohol, the Sufi mystics of Islam do not consider this injunction applicable to cannabis, which they insist reveals truth, rather than obscuring it.

Chapter 3, "Chinese Pharmacopoeia and the Golden Flower," marks a movement away from the religious and ritualistic uses of cannabis to its cultivation in China as a foodstuff, as a natural fiber, and as a healing agent by at least 1500 BCE—and likely much earlier. References to the plant occur frequently in Chinese literature, for instance, in the *Book of Songs*, *Bamboo Annals*, *Book of Odes*, as well as in some Daoists texts. With the exception of Chinese shamans adding it to teas and elixirs brewed for healing ceremonies, cannabis never gained wide acceptance as a psychoactive agent among the Han Chinese (although they made important contributions to the pharmacological understanding of marijuana as a treatment for a variety of ailments). On the other hand, Islamic Uyghurs in the Xinjiang region of northwest China, and some sects of Tibetan Vajrayāna Buddhism, still employ cannabis as a psychotropic agent.

With chapter 4, "Dagga Cults, Coptic Churches, and the Rastafari," we step out of the Middle East and onto the African continent to consider cannabis rituals in ancient Egypt and to ponder a cultural landscape in which members of cannabis cults (among the Khoikhoi, Zulus, Pygmies, and the Bena-Riamba) consume marijuana as a ritual sacrament and formidable medicine. The dagga cult meets Judeo-Christianity in the Rastafarian movement and gives birth to a religion that emphasizes communing with God and imbibing the hallowed plant in social, ceremonial, and recreational settings. The teachings of Jamaican-born Marcus Garvey, and the accession of Haile Selassie as emperor of Ethiopia, fired the zeal of the Rastafarians, and what they sometimes call "kali-weed" is now sanctified as a potent aid in the practice of spiritual introspection. As the inimitable Bob Marley once observed: the "herb make you meditate."[16]

Chapter 5, "Peak-Experiences and the Ineffable," contrasts mystical traditions separated by the abyss of time as a way to underscore the universal nature of self-transcendence. Eleusinian, Dionysian, and Mithraic Mysteries employed entheogens during secret rituals, while the ancient Scythians imbibed cannabis in funerary ceremonies and salvific rites. Similarly, Native American shamans utilized marijuana in a wide variety of healing contexts following its introduction during the sixteenth century. Our focus falls on the Cuna in Panama, the Cora of the Sierra Madre Occidental, and the Tepehuán of Vera Cruz (who use "Rosa Maria" in quasi-Christian ceremonies) in order to compare Native American ecstatic traditions with those found in the Western classical world.

In chapter 6, "Hashish Eaters, Hobbits' Leaf, and the Pantagruelion," we follow literary engagements with cannabis by writers in Europe and the United States from the Early Modern period (c. 1500–1800) into the mid-to-late-twentieth century. One-time Franciscan monk turned medical doctor, François Rabelais, celebrated marijuana as the queen of plants in his sixteenth-century masterwork *Gargantua and Pantagruel*. During the 1800s, an antibourgeois artist collective in Paris, known as the *Club des Hashischins* (Hash-eaters Club), chronicled a variety of cannabis-induced experiences along with the attributes of several other psychoactive substances. Counted among its members were such famed personages as Jacques-Joseph Moreau, Gustave Flaubert, Théophile Gautier, and Charles Baudelaire. In North America, Fitz Hugh Ludlow made solitary forays into the psychoactive properties of cannabis. By the turn of the twentieth century, W. B. Yeats and others would pick up where Ludlow and the hashish-eaters left off, and writers ranging from Allen Ginsberg to Terry Southern, Joan Didion to Don DeLillo, continued that investigatory work in the second half of the twentieth century. In extending our investigation of cannabis from its role in religion, culture, and medicine to secular literatures, a clandestine history of marijuana comes to light that lauds its consciousness-raising properties.

We undertake this far-ranging journey to better appreciate the prominence of cannabis in the cultural and religious history of humankind, and through that understanding to discover ways that the conscientious individual living in a country, state, or region with progressive marijuana laws might tap its potential as an agent of mental, physical, and spiritual well-being. Through a careful interrogation of core themes from a variety of religious and cultural traditions in which cannabis is found, my hope is to illuminate avenues for the responsible exploration of consciousness (which seems more important than ever in our digital age of distraction), and to provide guideposts for those aspiring to revitalize their minds and bodies by learning to abide in presence and a full awareness of the now.

Sacred Bliss summons the reader to explore the relationship between mental wholeness and physical healing by challenging traditional attitudes about cannabis—and encouraging casual users who might normally partake and watch a sports match at a local bar, go to a party, or chill out on the sofa instead to hone an attentive awareness that opens new dimensions of experience. For those living in chronic pain, enduring serious illness, or facing the inevitable cessation of the physical form, these pages hold the possibility of learning to disidentify with the body, and the repetitive patterns that govern so much of our habitual mentation, in order to recognize our true shared nature in the ground of being. As we learn to relinquish delusory notions of selfhood, what Sri Ramana Maharshi called "Being / Pure Consciousness / Bliss" unfolds before our very eyes and transforms our personal anguish into the kingdom of heaven. Where there was once a wasteland, a paradise is perceived in its place; this profound shift in perception allows one to live more fully from the creative center of being without competing, desiring, or regretting.

I

VEDĀNTA, SĀDHU PRIESTS, AND THE "LORD OF BHANG"

Bordered to the west by the Arabian Sea, the Indian Ocean to the south, the Bay of Bengal to the east, and the Himalayas and Hindu Kush to the north, the Indian subcontinent is distinguished by hilly plains traversed by lengthy rivers. The extensive river systems in the north encouraged early agricultural settlements, while dry woodlands provided shelter to reclusive tribes. Together these wetlands and forests offered a fecundity that for centuries succored locals, as well as the nomads, pilgrims, seers, traders, and troops who crisscrossed the continent.

From ancient times, the peoples of the Indian subcontinent derived considerable wealth from an abundance of natural resources (fruits, spices, medical herbs, and exotic animals) that were highly sought after in world markets. By exchanging that largess, Indian kings and merchants accumulated the fortunes upon which empires were built. The Roman thirst for Indian goods in the first century was so great that Pliny the Elder complained about capital draining out of the Roman economy as a result. The Mughal courts of the sixteenth and seventeenth centuries grew notoriously opulent, their plentiful wealth affording luxuries that would have bankrupted less affluent ruling dynasties. Stunningly, at the dawn of the Industrial Revolution in the eighteenth century, India's portion of global gross domestic product (GDP) nearly equaled Europe's 25 percent share.[1] That enormous body of wealth remained concentrated in a few hands—a phenomenon reinforced by a rigid caste system.

Commercial exchanges among members of the earliest communities led in time to cultural uniformity, and that collectivization gave rise to the first internal political rivalries.[2] Unlike the ancient civilizations in Mesopotamia, Egypt, Greece, and China—whose historical chronicles date from the third and second millenniums BCE—attempts at understanding the early peoples in India are stymied by a dearth of written records. Aside from the yet undeciphered carved seals found among the urban ruins of Mohenjo-Daro and Harappa (the Indus Valley Civilization), the earliest Indian script comes from Ashoka, the emperor who propagated Buddhism in the third century BCE. Tantalizing clues offered by those ornate seals, including human figures in apparent yogic or meditative postures, suggest an important continuity between early Vedic culture and the Hindu religion that emerged later. In that religious shift from animism to monism, cannabis found a sacred place as an entheogen.

At the height of its prosperity, between 2600 and 1900 BCE, the Indus Valley Civilization spanned 300,000 square miles in northwest India and Pakistan, and it included more than a thousand villages and townships. In fact, the urban culture of Indus Valley Civilization was more extensive than those in the empires in Mesopotamia and Egypt during the third century BCE.[3] Comparable in size to the cities of Ur in Mesopotamia and Memphis in Egypt, Mohenjo-Daro and Harappa featured buildings constructed from bricks formed to standard dimensions, and were set on streets that conformed to a grid-pattern, making Mohenjo-Daro and Harappa the world's first planned cities.[4] Mohenjo-Daro, for instance, flourished due to its ability to ensure the safe passage of goods and resources through land and water trading routes, to mobilize able workforces, and to effectively store crops (some of the city's largest buildings may have been dedicated granaries). Mohenjo-Daro even contained drainage for bathrooms and a municipal swimming pool (possibly important for public ritual absolutions or immersions).[5]

Two growing seasons sustained the peoples of the sprawling Indus Valley Civilization. Summer monsoons provided the water necessary to grow cannabis, grapes, dates, cotton, millet, and melons, while in the winter months wheat, oats, barley, lentils, beans, and jujube were harvested. They innovated an accurate system of weights and measures, adorned themselves with jewelry, and traded in the Persian Gulf region, as far as Afghanistan, and Mesopotamia (where Indus jewels, weights, and seals have been found).[6] As to its mode of governance, scholars assume that some kind of federation oversaw the villages, yet the early Indus Valley peoples built no great pyramids, grand temples, or alluring palaces. Nor did they leave behind loot-laden graves, defensive fortifications, or military weapons through which modern archeologists might better understand them.

Similarly, the causes for the disappearance of the Indus Valley Civilization eludes precise determination; in fact, we know little save that Indus scripts ceased to be produced during the early part of the second millennium BCE, and that they bear little resemblance to the Brahmi script that emerged nearly fifteen hundred years later with the Ashoka inscriptions. However, rather than being overrun by "Indo-Europeans," who composed the *Rig Veda* scripture, more likely the Indus Valley Civilization was contemporaneous with Vedic culture—or the Vedic tradition was its precursor.

In either case, the nineteenth-century notion of a massive invasion by lighter-skinned Aryans who displaced darker-complexioned aboriginals and drove them to the south has been discredited as a remnant of colonial ideology that justified racist policies and practices. Drought, and not outside aggressors, likely caused its deterioration.[7] Other possibilities for the decline and disappearance of the Indus Valley Civilization include deforestation due to over-grazing, natural disaster (earthquakes and river shifts), waterborne illnesses such as malaria and cholera, the rejection of central authority, and perhaps even the coming of foreigners from the northwest.[8] Quite probably, it was some combination of these factors.

Until the seals are deciphered, no clearer picture concerning those aspects of Indus Valley Civilization that are indigenous to the subcontinent, and those that come from outside, will be possible. Yet, a robust influence from Iran by the middle of the second millennium BCE onward gives way to Greek authority with the arrival of Alexander the Great in the third century BCE. Cannabis use in India precedes the advent of written record keeping and was firmly established long before the development of institutionalized religion—at a time when magic, mythology, healing, and sacrament blended seamlessly in shamanism, the oldest religious and spiritual tradition known to humankind (and one that exists to some extent among all pre-urban peoples). As such, it constitutes a major expression of human spirituality and healing, and we will therefore encounter the shamanic arts frequently in this spiritual history of cannabis.

Shaman healers and diviners often demonstrate receptivity to states of trance and ecstasy at a young age, and this feature of their personalities makes clear to other community members that they will follow a shamanistic path as they enter adulthood. Traditionally, shamans serve in many social capacities, including those of the physician, priest, oracle, diviner, magician, witch, midwife, herbalist, scientist, rhapsodist, storyteller, and mythmaker.[9] We best conceive shamanism as the cultivation of states of consciousness associated with mental and physical healing, as shamans treat all forms of illness attributed to physiological imbalances, psychological fragmentation, or possession by negative energies (or spirits). The medicinal plant herbs gathered and deployed by shamans are regarded as divine gifts from the natural world serving as catalysts for self-transformation.

Shamans have utilized cannabis to attain states of trance and meditation, and to suspend egoic grasping and rejecting, for thousands of years. Accessing those alternative states of consciousness moves the shaman or patient (sometimes both) out of the profane and into the sacred to effect recovery. A surprising internal coherency of practices and beliefs characterizes the shamanist endeavor across time and culture. In addition to deploying herbs like cannabis as one facet of holistic healing, shamans use the repetition of vocal and instrumental sound, manipulation of the breath, fasting, and prolonged sexual abstinence to help them enter trance states of consciousness.

Rather than dismissing such healing practices as primitive remnants of a prescientific worldview, the modern reader might envision the shamanistic pursuit of ecstasy as an act of spiritual surrender that simultaneously authenticates the individual self and the mystery of being. William A. Richards, an entheogen expert with the Johns Hopkins Bayview Medical Center, reminds us that shamans possess valuable knowledge to share, "not only concerning exotic herbs and concoctions, but also about techniques of navigating within consciousness and the spiritual interconnectedness of us all."[10] The loss of ordinary patterns of time and space and a radical realignment of perception, often culminating in some form of symbolic death and resurrection, are among the shifts in consciousness evoked by shamanic techniques of ecstasy.[11]

The ancient shamanic practices of journeying in search of a lost soul as a modality of healing appears in the *Rig Veda*, one of the oldest religious texts in any Indo-European language.[12] Composed around 1500

BCE and preserved orally until it was recorded in the first century, the *Rig Veda* is composed of a series of cryptic, discontinuous, and fragmentary hymns in verses that mostly refer to sacrifices, arcane rituals, and praises of various gods. Although the Hindus who succeeded the inhabitants of the Indus Valley Civilization did not identify with the material culture of their forbearers (and instead built grand temples to their deities), they venerated the *Vedas*. That scriptural tradition still provides ascetic seekers with a rationale for the rejection of cherished customs and worldly values, and it also sanctifies the ingestion of entheogens, including cannabis, to induce peak-experiences.

Taken together, the four Vedas (the *Rig*, *Yajur*, *Sama*, and *Atharva*) represent a diversified but continuous religious tradition of approximately a thousand years in duration. Each Veda contains four parts: *Samhitas* ("Collections" of mantras and praises to God), *Brahmanas* ("Sacred Expositions" on rituals and sacrifices), *Aranyakas* ("Forest Books" on proper ceremonial worship), and *Upanishads* ("Sitting Near" a master to receive philosophical and spiritual teachings). The term "Veda" denotes a state of "knowledge, knowing, or seeing," while "Vedānta" indicates its culmination in peak religious experiences of nonduality (codified in subsequent religious texts, such as the *Brahma Sutras*, *Upanishads*, and the *Bhagavad Gītā*).[13] In this way, the polytheistic worldview held by sages (rishis) in the *Rig Veda* period was gradually supplanted by an emphasis on the nondual nature of reality in classical Hinduism.

In the early Vedic *Samhitas*, heroic visionary rishis engage various gods and powers thought to pervade the world in a quest for self-transcendent experiences assisted by ascetic practices and the ingestion of a mysterious plant elixir called "soma" (that may have included cannabis). The *Rig Veda*, a book of kings and sages, narrates the rise of a great civilization in the northern Indus Valley, and it includes discussions of creation, nature, women, pastoral life, animals (particularly cows and horses), and death. It also memorializes the victories of Vedic priests and kings who made the kingdom of Bharata into a spiritual realm of yoga, tapas (asceticism), and self-realization.[14]

The one thousand verses that make up the *Rig Veda* provide specific instructions for priests regarding the proper conduct of ritual sacrifices, and they contain a variety of incantations and magic spells believed to have powerful repercussions in the natural world. Since the gods were thought to owe their divine positions, and very existences, to the sacrificial act—the highly complicated ritualistic system, codified in the *Rig Veda*, furthered the machinations of a priestly class eager to advance its own agenda by making important sacrifices ends in themselves, rather than means for propitiating gods and acquiring ritual power.

The chief deities of the *Rig Veda* were personified as forces of nature (sun, fire, wind, sky, rain), and they were the foci of regular ritual sacrifices—as were other principal gods, including Varuṇa (guardian of sacred laws and the divine order), Prajapati (lord of creatures and the primeval person whose dismemberment creates the phenomenal world and the four castes), Agni (the fire god who consumes the sacrificial offerings and conveys them to the gods), Yama (the god of death who looks after the souls of the departed), and Soma (the god of a tonic of eternal life pressed from a psychedelic plant). [15] According to one myth, Indra (the god of war and weather) is borne to heaven by an eagle, and he returns to earth with the soma plant for the mutual benefit of human beings and the gods. [16] Book 8 of the *Rig Veda* contains the following enigmatic hymn celebrating the ecstatic effects of the soma potion:

> We have drunk the Soma; we have become immortal; we have gone to the light; we have found the gods. What can hatred and the malice of a mortal do to us now, O immortal one?
>
> When we have drunk you, O drop of Soma, be good to our heart, kind as a father to his son, thoughtful as a friend to a friend. Far-famed Soma, stretch out our lifespan so that we may live.
>
> The glorious drops that I have drunk set me free in wide space. You have bound me together in my limbs as thongs bind a chariot. Let the drops protect me from the foot that stumbles and keep lameness away from me.
>
> Inflame me like a fire kindled by friction; make us see far; make us richer, better. For when I am intoxicated with you, Soma, I think myself rich. Draw near and make us thrive. [17]

The *Soma Mandala* that makes up the ninth book of the *Rig Veda* features more than one hundred similar dedications to *soma pavamāna*, the purifying soma, as a means of winning "heavenly light" and "all felicities." The employment of entheogens continues in modern Hinduism, although milder psychoactive plants such as cannabis have replaced the highly psychedelic soma brew as a stimulus for religious experience.

The fire sacrifices central to early Vedic ritual also have correlates in the Mithraic and Zoroastrian traditions discussed in the next chapter. Translations of Vedic fire hymns offer a window to a multidimensional animistic world where all organisms, objects, and even abstract principles are regarded as enlivened by spirits. In the following hymn to *Agni* (the god of fire who transmutes sacrificial offerings), note the central role of fire to proper worship, along with the cryptic nature of the verses:

1. You, O Agni (god Fire) are Varuṇa when you are born. You become Mitra (god Courtship) when you are kindled. In you, O son of strength, are all gods. You are Indra for the pious mortal.

2. You become Aryaman, in that you belong to maidens, you bear this secret name, O self-mighty one. Like a friend well-accepted they anoint you with ghee, since you make a married couple concordant.

3. Unto your glory the followers of Indra adorn themselves, when your beautiful, wondrous birth takes place. What was set down as the highest footsteps of Vishnu, with that you (Fire) guard the secret name of the cows. [18]

Esoteric passages such as this one from the *Rig Veda* shed light on an animistic belief system that provided a mythic framework through which control was sought over all creatures, things, powers, and even abstract principles—in short, all "spirits"—through incantations and magic rites.

Evident also from such passages is an evolution of Vedic Brahmanism out of shamanism, for all shamanistic traditions include some form of botanicals to bestow access to the divine (usually consumed in conjunction with ritual acts such as prayer, mantra, and meditation). [19] Like the shamans before them, village Brāhman priests prayed for individuals, ensured the collective welfare by warding off spirits, cured diseases, helped defeat enemies, and brought wealth and prosperity to their communities. Ensuring peace and harmony, and providing a path for the inward development of human consciousness beyond the ego, were also credited to Brahmanic rites—and out of them grew yoga, as well as the belief in individual paths to salvation. [20]

Yet, over time, the elaborate rites of nature-worship in the *Rig Veda* became the exclusive dispensation of powerful aristocrats (who used them to secure wealth, social prestige, and to mediate social issues regarding the welfare of the kingdom). In the emergence of that social hierarchy, we find the origin of the Hindu caste system: priests (Brāhmans or Brahmins) who recited Vedic mantras; warriors (Kshatriya) who fought enemies; merchants (Vaishya) who fabricated and traded goods; and laborers (Shudra) who provided the toil upon which the wealth of others was built. An "untouchable" caste (Dalits) handled dead bodies, cleaned sewers, and dispensed with the waste products of human civilization.

The *Atharva Veda* represents a backlash against the aristocratic elitism of the *Rig Veda* cult, and it most directly preserves ancient shamanistic rites dealing with village concerns, individual well-being, and the use of magic hymns to "control" all elements of nature.[21] Recited in religious masses composed of simpler ceremonies and sacrifices than those prescribed in the *Rig Veda*, the hymns in the *Atharva Veda* include the imprecations, blessings, prayers, and magical spells of the type discoverable in popular superstitions at all times, and in all countries. A belief in their efficacy encouraged adherents to appease the gods and secure their protecting favor through the recitation of mantras thought to remedy ills and mend mental and physical wounds. Compiled sometime later than the *Rig Veda* but likely before 1000 BCE, the *Atharva Veda* is especially relevant to our survey, as it contains some of the oldest direct references to the ritualistic use of cannabis in the world.

For example, book 2 of the *Atharva Veda* features a hymn to win protection from injury, ensure good health, and bring prosperity, and it is rendered effectual by wearing a charmed amulet. In that incantation, cannabis is lauded as a panacea for rheumatism and a variety of other ills— and it also receives praise for its special ability to ward off demons! While somewhat obscure to the contemporary nonspecialist, this passage illustrates the magical properties that ritually sanctified objects were understood to possess. One section of hymn four reads:

This [amulet of a thousand powers] overcomes illness, this chases the greedy fiends away: May this our panacea, may herbs save us from distress.
With the herb that brings delight, Amulet given by the Gods, We in the conflict overcome illness and all Rākshasas [demonic beings].
May Cannabis and Jangida [herbs] preserve me from Vishkandha [illness],—that Brought to us from the forest, this sprung from the saps of husbandry.
This Amulet destroys the might of magic and malignity: So may victorious herbs prolong the years we have to live.[22]

Many hymns in the *Atharva Veda* reinforce the healing potential of hallowed plants, such as soma, *darbha*, and *kuśa*. Practitioners of this ancient religious tradition utilized cannabis as a medicinal herb, and because of its centrality to charms and spells, cannabis was regarded a "sacred grass" for its power to vanquish sickness, despair, and calamity. In book 11 of the *Atharva Veda*, we find these suggestive lines affirming those strengths:

> To the five kingdoms of the plants [that] Soma rules as Lord we speak.
> *Darbha*, hemp, barley, mighty power: may these deliver us from woe.
> To demons and fierce fiends we speak, to Holy Genii, Fathers, Snakes,
> And to the hundred deaths and one: may these deliver us from woe. [23]

In this excerpt, the god Soma animates the plant world and rules over it as sovereign—and cannabis, *darbha* grass, and barley are singled out as exemplars of gifts offered to humanity in order to sustain life, remedy illness, and deflect evil forces.

Although hymns to the god Soma appear frequently in the *Atharva Veda* (as they do in the *Rig Veda*), the precise ingredients of that psychedelic potion bearing his name are subject to ongoing debate. Scholars such as Christian Rätsch,[24] S. Mahdihassan,[25] and Robert Clark and Mark Merlin[26] argue that soma contained a mixture of *Cannabis indica* and *Ephedra gerardiana*. Whether the fly-agaric mushroom (*Amanita muscaria*) that grows in the northern mountains was added to these two primary ingredients, or was itself the sacred soma plant,[27] we may never know. Indisputably, however, its ingestion during religious ceremonies was a means of inducing peak-experiences in ritual participants. More generally, the hymns to the god Soma in the *Vedas* point toward the veneration of certain plants for their ability to put religious seekers in direct contact with the divine. The lightweight carts (in which harvested soma plants were transported to be pressed), the containers into which that elixir was poured, and even the priests who presided over the ritual ceremonies are all described in the *Atharva Veda*. In such passages, the god Indra is the "Lord of Soma," the chief guzzler of the revered beverage—and he regularly overdoses on it.

As later generations appropriated the *Rig Veda*, *Atharva Veda*, and other Vedic scriptures, the transition from Vedic Brahmanism to Hinduism happened almost imperceptibly (for certain "Hinduistic" elements were already present in Vedic society, as some images on the Indus

Valley seals suggest). Philosophically speaking, Brahman (to be distinguished from Brāhman priests and their rituals) came to represent more
than the power of mantras recited at soma rites in which choir singers
accompanied staged performances by the priests; Brahman became a basic cosmic principle in the *Atharva Veda* and evolved into a belief in the
fundamental unity of the universe. That transition marks an important
shift from ritual (where the sound of mantras and hymns were typically
given more significance than their oft-obscure meanings) to more general
speculative philosophical questions regarding the nature of the universe.[28] In the wake of that evolution, some Vedic gods suffered diminu-
tion as others grew in stature (an organic process that continued into the
Puranic Ages). Indra, for example, retained his popularity but lost his
status as leader of the gods. Conversely, Shiva and Vishnu (along with
their female consorts) take exceptional positions in what became the Hindu trinity (trimūrti).[29]

In that triune, the god Brahmā (distinct from the cosmic principle
Brahman) becomes creator, Vishnu preserver, and Shiva destroyer of the
cosmos. Working together, they bring forth all material manifestations,
allow them to go through their transformations, and welcome them back
to nonbeing. In this manner, they sustain the universe in exquisite balance. The truth of the transience of the material world is symbolized in
the figure of the Lord of the Dance, the cosmic dancer Shiva Nataraja,
who beats the drum of time in his uppermost right hand, which summons
forth the material world from nonbeing, thereby giving all things their
temporary physical aspect. In his uppermost left hand, he brandishes the
fire by which all material creation is forthwith destroyed. The figure of
Shiva Nataraja makes symbolic the gradual transition from animism to
monism in Indian thought, a point that is central to this study—and not
simply because Shiva is known to be as fond of cannabis, as Indra is of
soma.

Out of that monistic belief in the existence of a single Supreme Being
sprung an uncompromising nondualistic worldview in which all material
manifestations in the cosmos ultimately dissolve—erasing bifurcations of
self and other, god and humankind, along with them. The deities of the
trimūrti (and the other gods) were reconceived as manifestations of a
single principle by which the whole universe might be known. This transition from ritual concerns to philosophical questions about the nature of
reality led directly to the theory of Ātman (self or breath) in Hindu

thought. Distinguishable from the physical body, Ātman constitutes the basic reality of a person, and it endures after death. To truly understand the core principles that propel cannabis culture in India, this admittedly arcane religious philosophy requires unpacking.

During the last half of the first millennium, the basic creed of the later *Upanishads* asserted that Brahman dwells within every human being as the Ātman. Thus, Ātman and Brahman were made one, and so the mystical expression to "become Brahman" denotes a merging of the self with the infinite. Through a unitive experience of this doctrinal truth, egoic constructions of self and the world are stripped away to reveal (often in a flash) one's true nature as unconditioned, eternal, and wholly free. When the self (Ātman) becomes aware of its identity with that ultimate principle, it is released from bondage—which is called moksha, or emancipation.

The emphasis on attaining firsthand experiential knowledge of reality by way of unitive perception finds voice in the *Īshā Upanishad*, which offers this wise counsel regarding nonduality:

> The Lord is enshrined in the hearts of all.
> The Lord is the supreme Reality.
> Rejoice in him through renunciation.
> Covet nothing. All belongs to the Lord.[30]

In addition to pointing toward the truth of nonduality, this passage emphasizes a tradition of renunciation dating back to the *Rig Veda*, one that sanctions leaving family, wealth, and all manner of bodily comforts behind in pursuit of self-annihilation and spiritual rebirth. Itinerant cannabis-smoking Hindu mendicants, known as Sādhus, illustrate one outcome of making moksha the goal of human life—only they do not wait for old age to seek liberation, as traditionally prescribed in the four stages of Hindu life (the *ashrama*).

The ascetic impulse in Hinduism finds voice in those four phases in human life (the young student, adult householder, middle-aged forest dweller, and elderly renouncer). In the fleeting days of youth, one should study, but never fail to meet the familial responsibilities that adulthood invariably brings. In middle age, one retires to the forest after family obligations are dispatched. In old age, moving no matter how reluctantly toward death, one forsakes material wealth, discards all remaining biases, and lives austerely in accordance with dharma (duty, law, truth) until the body is finished. In this fourth stage of life, moksha is put within reach, for instead of clinging to a bodily existence that one will soon be leaving, a connection which only increases suffering, the elder Hindu strives to break all attachments to the transitory world while still alive.

Although this vision of existence may sound morose to some readers, it contains a lovely acknowledgment of the natural processes of birth, life, and death. Broadly speaking, liberation from suffering is the goal of all Indian philosophies and techniques of meditation. Indian religious literature employs tropes of binding, fettering, or captivity—of forgetting, sleep, or unknowing—to depict the unawakened mind. Yet, release from bondage and rending of the veil are just two metaphors associated with awakening, remembering, and seeing.[31] For the individual who transcends duality and learns to perceive "all creatures in himself," the self is discovered everywhere indivisible and untouched by sin (a state of separation).

In the *Māndūkya Upanishad*, this "fourth state" of supraconsciousness is deemed the "supreme goal of life" because it represents the realization of infinite peace and love. The spirit of this vision is remarkably close to other mystics who have testified to religious experiences.[32] We recall from the introduction that Abraham Maslow found peak-experiences to be universal occurrences that culminate in the collapse of distinctions between self and other, a gracious dissolution in feelings of profound gratitude and connectedness to all beings. Eknath Easwaran's luminous translation of the *Shvetāshvatara Upanishad* gives elegant expression to the process of interpenetration that comes with the erasure of dichotomies of self and other (Ātman and Brahman) in the mind of the highly realized mystic:

> The Lord of Love, omnipresent, dwelling
> In the heart of every living creature,
> All mercy, turns every face to himself.
>
> He is the supreme Lord who through his grace
> Moves people to him in their own hearts.
> He is the light that shines forever.
>
> He is the inner Self all who is
> Hidden like a little flame in the heart.
> Only by the stilled mind can he be known.
> Those who realize him become immortal.[33]

This reference to immortality should not be interpreted to mean that the bodily form shall abide forever, but instead that the true essence (Ātman) in oneself *is* the imperishable, eternal, everlasting Brahman. By learning to sever identification with a view of the self as bodily form, or worse as a stream of egoic thought patterns, the spiritual aspirant opens new vistas of experience, which are at once self-transcendent and utterly grounded in the ever-present Now.

In the *Bhagavad Gītā* (*Song of God*), the heart of the Hindu epic *Mahābhārata*, Lord Krishna grants the warrior Arjuna a peak-experience of nonduality that engenders B-cognition. The *Mahābhārata*, which reaches final form in the fourth century, recounts a dynastic family struggle between the Kauravas (sons of Dhritarashtra and descendants of Kuru) and the virtuous Pandavas (sons of Pandu). The intrigue begins when Dhritarashtra invites the Pandavas to a game of dice, a contest that they are honor-bound to accept. Unbeknownst to the Pandavas, the dice are loaded; they lose, forfeit their kingdom of Indraprastha to the Kauravas, and embark on a thirteen-year period of exile—at the end of which the Pandavas are to regain rights of leadership. Years later, when the Kauravas refuse to restore Indraprastha to its just rulers, war becomes inevitable between the cousins.

The prospect of combat also provides a poignant reminder of the truth found in the Ātman equals Brahman formulation, and the battle that ensues epitomizes a broader struggle between dharma and *adharma* (injustice, unrighteousness) in the world. As the Pandavan and Kauravan armies face off on the battlefield at Kurukshetra for a pitched eighteen-day struggle between relatives and close relations, the Pandava leader Arjuna gives voice to grave doubts concerning the wisdom of fighting cousins, teachers, and other relations amassed on the frontline for the sake of worldly power and the wealth that accompanies a prosperous kingdom. Those doubts make the thoughtful warrior incapable of action on the field of battle, and so he turns to Krishna as a wartime counselor—choosing him over the entire Kaurava army (replete with their magic weapons).

Krishna will not bear arms or enter the fray, but Arjuna's shrewd decision to value wise counsel over brute force demonstrates that he possesses an integrity lacking in his Kuru adversaries. In his unwillingness to fight, Arjuna clings to a popular, but ultimately unnuanced, understanding of karma and dharma. Arjuna believes that slaying fathers, grandsires, uncles, brothers, and their sons would bring negative conse-

quences upon himself, his family, and the kingdom. Entering the deadly
mêlée to gain a kingdom would also seem to transgress the codes of
dharma—a moral lapse that would inhibit his ability to reach moksha in
this life or the following ones.

His concerns seem justified, for according to Hindu belief an individual born into a particular caste remains duty-bound to it. Hindu priests
have an obligation to protect the scriptures, warriors to defend their com-
rades, merchants to ply their trades, and workers to labor at a variety of
necessary tasks. Through adherence to the responsibilities of dharma corresponding to caste, one could generate enough positive karma to effect a
higher reincarnation—a conception that helped to rationalize India's
highly tiered class system. Moksha (a goal for all Hindus that ends the
transmigration of the soul) was considered easiest to achieve in the priestly caste, due to Brahmanic proximity to, and fluency with, sacred scriptures.

While racked with concern about the karmic consequences of killing
kinfolk, teachers, and friends for personal gain, Arjuna remains unwilling
to fight. Yet the moral calculus of the *Bhagavad Gītā* favors the virtuous
actor and punishes the wicked in thought or deed, and Arjuna's selection
of wisdom (Krishna) over military might (the Kaurava army) presages the
victory of the Pandavas in spite of the superior forces of their foes. Arjuna's misgivings, therefore, spring from a misinterpretation of karma,
caste, and duty. In consulting Krishna for a solution to his quandary (who
unbeknownst to the warrior is an avatar of Vishnu), Arjuna gains an
esoteric understanding of karmic law.

Krishna explains to the doubt-ridden warrior that desireless action will
not generate karma. For this reason, Arjuna need only to act in battle as if
he were doing so by proxy, in another's stead, to avoid enslavement to a
karmic circuit of cause and effect, and reincarnation through endless
rounds of birth and death.[34] As a member of the Kshatriya caste, Arjuna
must defend his kingdom from all threats, but by following the path of
selfless action, by fighting impersonally without passion or attachment—
indifferent to the fruits of his actions—Arjuna may remain pure of karmic
taint while on the field of battle.

The revelation of how to relinquish attachment to all actions in the
world—*and yet to still act in it*, comes in the form of a spectacular vision
of the unity of reality, a peak-experience that Krishna discloses to Arjuna
(along with the reader). In it, all apparent dualities (of creation and de-

struction, life and death, self and other) are discovered to be the result of arbitrary intellectual distinctions. Krishna explains:

> Of what is not there is no becoming;
> Of what there is no ceasing to be:
> For the boundary-line between these two
> Is seen by men who see things as they really are.

> Indestructible alone is That—know this—
> By which the whole universe was spun.
> No one at all can bring destruction
> On This which passes not away.

> Finite, they say, are these bodies
> Indwelt by an eternal embodied soul,
> A soul indestructible, incommensurable.
> Fight then, O scion of the Bharata clan!

> Who thinks that he can be a slayer,
> Who thinks he is slain,
> Both these lack right knowledge:
> He slays not, is not slain.

> Never is he born nor dies:
> Never did he come to be, nor will he never come to be again:
> Unborn, eternal, everlasting he—primeval:
> He is not slain when the body is no more.[35]

Here, Krishna imparts the highest truth of nonduality (*Advaita*, "not-two") to Arjuna: the realization that his own imagined separateness from Brahman is a false idea resulting from an wrongful equation of the self (Ātman) with the temporal body, rather than with one's true nature (as Brahman). The teaching "thou art that" (*tat tvam asi*) powerfully express-es the unitive truth of Arjuna's realization—and it has provided reassu-rance to individuals suffering serious illness, harsh adversity, or the de-mise of the body.

By making evident the ground of being, as a unity beyond all bifurca-tions and oppositions, Krishna proclaims the end of dualistic perception, and in prophetic language suggestive of the soma rites, he summons the reader to awaken to the all-encompassing unity of the divine. He declares:

> I am the rite, the sacrifice,
> I am the offering, the herb.
> I am the mantra and the *ghee*,

I am fire and oblation;

The father of this universe,
its mother and grandfather, too;
object of knowledge, soma-strainer,
sacred OM, the three chief *Vedas*;

I am the way, the Lord, the witness;
abode, refuge, companion;
origin, death, and all between;
sepulcher and treasure horde.

I radiate heat, Arjuna,
I hold back rain and let it go,
I am immortal life and death,
I am being and nonbeing.[36]

Because ratiocination is blind to the fundamental oneness of reality, this splendid visionary experience bestowed by Krishna rouses the great archer to the field of battle. Through a direct understanding that there is no killer or killed, Arjuna intuitively apprehends the correct course of action for a member of the warrior caste who has dropped off all aspirations for the fruits of his actions—and he enters the bout.

Arjuna's salvation comes in discerning that no distinction between self and other remains tenable to one who identifies with the undifferentiated energy that flows through all things, rather than material forms constantly in flux (which are its manifestations). The true yogi transcends all contraries and unites life and death, being and nonbeing, into a primordial nonduality.[37] The mendicant Sādhus who bring this chapter to a close take these Hindu doctrines of renunciation and nondualism to an extreme in their quest for salvation, and they make cannabis an integral aspect of that pursuit. As we shall see, theirs is a meaningful response to core Hindu teachings.

The *Katha Upanishad* asserts, for instance, that a person "who knows the soundless, odorless, tasteless, intangible, formless, deathless, supernatural undecaying, beginningless, endless, unchangeable Reality, springs out of the mouth of death."[38] Nothing—certainly not the pursuit of material comforts that the postindustrial world values so highly—is more important to the spiritually minded Hindu than realizing, in this very life, the basic fact that self and God are one. Sādhus direct their spiritual vision inward and ground it in a firsthand apprehension of the unity of all being. They also draw inspiration from Vedic descriptions of munis (seers or silent ones).

Book 10 of the *Rig Veda* describes munis as wearing "long loose locks" and being "girdled with the wind," meaning that they went about largely naked as an outward sign of their renunciation. These mendicants follow only "the wind's swift course and go where the Gods have gone before," spurning all enticements to worldliness that might hinder their journey to moksha. Munis in the *Rig Veda* fly through the atmosphere looking down detachedly "upon all varied forms" of life, and in this way they are "made associate in the holy work of every God."[39] Munis, who stand firmly outside of the Vedic mainstream, long suffered marginalization by a priestly elite whose highly structured ceremonial rituals held no place for soiled and naked wanderers who rejected ceremonial pomp. In time, however, Brāhman priests adopted many ascetic practices of the munis, including fasting, meditation, celibacy, ritual forms of exercise and breathing, and self-flagellation for rites such as the soma sacrifice.

Readers familiar with Buddhism will recall that Siddhārtha Gautama experimented with every form of Indian asceticism available to him in the fourth or fifth century BCE before formulating a creed of the middle way between extremes of deprivation and indulgence. Notwithstanding that path of moderation championed by the Buddha, asceticism as an ideal persisted in Indian religious traditions (most notably among the Jains and Ājīvakas). In the eastern kingdoms of the sixth century, Indian ascetics and renunciates (*sramanas*) wore their hair matted as an emblematic statement of protest against the materialistic values held by rulers, merchants, and the general population. They spurned the authority of Brāhman priests and their emphasis on the continuance of ancestor cults, and the caste system, which placed Brāhmans in the top position.[40]

Sādhus, who are found all over India, therefore practice a form of asceticism that dates back to at least 1500 BCE when munis wandered naked (or symbolically in orange rags) and kept noble silence. Sādhu doctrines of release by way of experiential knowledge draw inspiration from ancient seers, who like tribal shamans or "witch doctors" entered states of ecstasy that transcended the limitations of the physical body. Sādhus eschew what most Hindus hold dear and openly flout the laws, customs, and taboos of Indian culture. Like the munis, some Sādhus become forest hermits or itinerate beggars and preachers, while others practice harsh penances or sit quietly in meditation.[41] Spiritual teachers (gurus) initiate aspiring Sādhus who demonstrate a profound desire to sever all worldly ties, including those of family and caste. In this manner, young Sādhus essentially move directly to the fourth stage of renunciation in the *ashrama*.

Many Sādhus find homes in welcoming ashrams or remote caves, while others move about continually and congregate around holy sites and funeral bonfires (where the transition between life and death provides the raw material for their rejection of social mores). They unabashedly transgress taboos, wear little or no clothing, cover themselves in funerary ash from human bodies, perform rites at cremations where mortality is always on display, and beg or scavenge for food. Sādhus also cast off restrictions regarding who they worship; they might devote themselves to the deities (or avatars) of Shiva, Vishnu, or Shakti—the primordial female energy of the universe. No matter which deities Sādhus choose to adore, they do so with an understanding that all Hindu gods and goddesses are ultimately one in Brahman. They undertake mendicant lives of deprivation in full awareness of the physical hardships that come with it, and they welcome them in a spirit of self-surrender.

Like other ascetics who live on the periphery of Indian society, many Sādhus are yogins who possess considerable knowledge about herbal medicines (including marijuana). As contemporary ideological descendants of Vedic munis, Sādhus are intriguing for reasons other than their keenness for cannabis and unconventional customs: they offer a vivid illustration of one spiritual response to the uncompromising nonduality of the *Upanishads* and the *Gītā*. Legendary for smoking copious amounts of ganja and occasionally making a meal out of a burning human corpse, their intimacy with death is sometimes symbolized in begging bowls fashioned from human skulls found along the river Ganges (where floating funeraries return burning bodies to sacred waters). Handcrafted ritual items, such as skull begging bowls, serve as formidable reminders of a shared human fate—with each meal.

In hopes that their unorthodox way of life makes sense as a reasoned response to ancient Indian ideals of renunciation and the philosophical development of the doctrine of nonduality, this chapter ends with an especially interesting Sādhu sect, the Aghori, who make sport of disobeying cultural and religious proscriptions. In fact, Aghori Sādhus seek to obliterate all distinctions between the pure and impure, and as proof of attaining such a perception, they might consume human bile in that spirit of unity. Indeed, theirs is a deep-seated rejection of all things deemed either "sacred" or "profane" by less ascetically inclined Hindus. [42] As one might gather, most Aghori Sādhus have no compunction about eating meat, drinking alcohol, or smoking ganja from chillum pipes in public. Indeed, cannabis is thought to assist Sādhu mendicants in their goal of finding oblivion in the grace of God.

While some Sādhu practices might seem extreme, they are far from the only Hindu sect to employ cannabis (in the form of bhang, ganja, or charas) as an integral part of religious practice, ritual, and ceremony. The Hindu god Shiva is extremely fond of hemp products, an affection that earned him the soubriquet the "Lord of Bhang" (a correlate to Indra as the "Lord of Soma"). From the proclivities exhibited by both gods, we realize that the peoples of the Indian subcontinent have long understood that plants such as cannabis are useful tools in exploring consciousness. As evidence of the serious religious intention with which devotees approach cannabis as a vehicle for religious experience, marijuana remains a socially permissible part of many religious and cultural events in India, a primary herb in traditional Ayurvedic medicine, as well as a "food for the gods" worthy of sacrificial offering.

Because it is widely known that wandering Sādhu ascetics and other renunciates rely on cannabis, layman gain merit by giving gifts of the plant to those who have forsaken all possessions in their quest for truth. Sādhu and Hindu mendicants crossing the Himalayas to visit holy shrines and temples associated with Shiva, for instance, consume cannabis for a variety of reasons: as an aid in meditation, to ease the difficulty of living a harsh itinerant lifestyle, as a means of camaraderie among fellow ascetics, and for the multifold benefits of cannabis as a medicine. [43] At holy festivals such as the *Shivaratri* and the *Kumbha Mela*, bhang is consumed as a holy drink to awaken inner light—and ganja is burned and exhaled in abundant offerings to Shiva. For Shivites, smoking marijuana provides a means by which to offer thanks to Lord Shiva, frequently depicted holding bowls filled with healing herbs, for its salutary effects. So sacrosanct are the numerous forms of cannabis ingestion in India that its secular use for recreational purposes is regarded as profane.

Of course, the prominent place of cannabis in religious ritual and medicine is not limited to the ancient world or to the Indian subcontinent; comparable engagements with marijuana can be discovered across Asia, Africa, and the Caribbean. Cannabis serves not only as an important sacrament for Hindu mendicants, but also for Islamic Sufis, Chinese Daoists, members of African dagga cults, and Jamaican Rastafarians.[44] Prior to the eighth and ninth centuries in India (when the arrival of Islam meant prohibitions against intoxicants such as alcohol), the consumption of hemp drinks was even more widespread. Nonetheless, to this day on the Indian continent, ganja is smoked, charas resin inhaled, and bhang formed into small balls and eaten (or consumed as *thandai*) in a variety of religious and spiritual ritual contexts.[45] Leaving those traditions behind, we now turn to Zoroastrian shamans in Persia, follow Sufi mystics in the wake of Islam, and investigate a secret "green language" used by Arabic poets and writers to extoll the virtues of cannabis.

2

SHAMANS, SUFIS, AND THE "GREEN MAN"

For thousands of years, cannabis has provided human beings in the Middle East with a nutritious food source, a safe medicinal herb, and a strong natural fiber for practical applications such as rope and fabric making. This long-standing relationship between humankind and cannabis, reaching far back into prehistory, points toward a co-evolutionary process whereby that plant found manifold ways to make itself desirable to human beings, especially in producing chemicals to alter consciousness in positive ways. By appealing thus to the body and mind, cannabis borrowed human locomotion to ensure its cultivation around the region, and eventually the globe. [1]

On the Iranian plateau, surrounded by the Hindu Kush to the east, the Mesopotamian Plain to the west, the Caspian Sea to the north, and the Persian Gulf to the south, a group of Indo-Iranian peoples emerged some six millennia ago. Most likely, the ceremonial, ritualistic, and recreational use of cannabis began in this part of the world and then spread eastward into Asia following established trade routes—before moving westward to Egypt, across Africa, and later into Europe. Ancient Indo-Iranian peoples made sacrifices to a variety of gods and goddesses, employed a priestly class to oversee those rites, and created a stratified social system that sustained a lifestyle built around the plow. In addition to tending livestock, they raised horses, which allowed them to roam over vast distances in search of resources. They spoke a Proto–Indo-European language that more than five thousand years ago diverged into many branches (including Germanic, Italic, Hellenic, and Indo-Iranian).

Due to the remarkable similarity of the Avestan language and Vedic Sanskrit, comparative analysis of Old Avestan scriptures with the *Rig Veda* is proving invaluable in reconstructing a shared Indo-Iranian heritage (out of which both cultures evolved separately). Iranian rituals and reforms to the Vedic pantheon, for example, shed more light on Indo-Iranian cultural beliefs than do Sanskrit sources alone.[2] This shared heritage helps to account for correspondences between Vedic religious texts and the *Gāthā* sections of the *Avesta* (or *Zend-Avesta*), the sacred book of Zoroastrianism. Preserved orally in the Avestan language, but compiled and recorded much later, the *Avesta* contains legal, literary, and liturgical writings (hymns, prayers, founding myths, and invocations)—in addition to collations of religious law, mythical tales, litanies, hymns, short prayers, and praise songs for recitation during calendrical ceremonies in which plant and animal sacrifices were shared with the divinities.

Ritual performances based on the *Avesta* scripture transmuted offerings to the gods and featured dramatic reenactments of founding myths, thereby transforming sacred stories into vehicles by which human beings co-participated in the divine act of creation. In their creation myths, plant and animal sacrifices put the universe in motion in seven stages.[3] Avestan deities maintained a cosmic order based on oppositional forces, and they associated supernatural beings with phenomena in the natural world. Like their Indian counterparts, the ancient Iranians venerated sky and earth gods and goddesses, worshiped ancestors (who offered protection when properly honored), and participated in cults of fire and water. Iranian priests served as libation pourers, keepers of sacred fires, and preservers of powerful mantras (chants, charms, and spells). Ecclesiastics, believed to possess magic powers and knowledge of immortality, sometimes accompanied warriors on raids to ensure their success.[4]

Similarities such as these to the *Rig Veda* should not surprise, for the *Gāthā* sections of the *Avesta* are contemporaneous with it, and the geographical horizon for both texts is northern Iran, eastern Afghanistan, and northwestern Pakistan. The Zoroastrian deity Mithra exhibits some of the same attributes as the gods *Mitrá* and Varuṇa in the *Rig Veda*. These shared conventions are markers of the fluency of exchange among peoples in the ancient Indo-Iranian world, and they provide further evidence of the geographical and cultural proximity of the Vedic and Avestan religions (during a joint Indo-Iranian period). At some point, a rivalry between the groups emerged and inaugurated a process of scriptural transmission during which some features of early Vedic culture were preserved by Iran Zarathustrans while others were reformed or altogether rejected, such as the practice of raiding cattle and the worship of Vedic *devas*.[5]

The prophet Zoroaster (Zarathustra) forever transformed that shared Indo-Iranian tradition by proclaiming the preeminence of the god Ahura Mazdā—while diminishing the importance of competing deities and modifying or abandoning certain ritual practices. He reimagined Ahura Mazdā as a unitive creative force (whereas before him divine agency was diffuse or unattributable), and as a consequence Zoroaster is often credited with innovating monotheism. Even so, there is good reason to remain leery of a progressive notion of religious history that envisions monotheism as a more "advanced" stage of human spiritual development than polytheism or shamanism—since monotheism often emerges as a consequence of imposition and the consolidation of power by a particular group.

From the *Gāthās*, the part of the *Zend-Avesta* thought to preserve the words of the tradition's founder, we gather that Zoroaster was a camel manager belonging to the priestly class who lived sometime around the fifth century BCE.[6] He created important roles for himself as an interpreter of religious commandments and bestower of spiritual instruction. Out of these vocations sprung a set of ethics that emphasized the human capacity to choose between good and evil forces in the world. That cosmic dualism became embedded in the Zoroastrian notion of time, envisioned as linear rather than cyclic, at the end of which a great battle between the forces of light (benevolence) and darkness (malevolence) concluded with the triumph of the good.

Zoroaster believed that an individual's fate was determined by free will, and not heavenly mandate. After the death of the human body, the soul was believed to make its way to a river of fire where the god Mithra—flanked by two celestial beings holding aloft the scales of justice—judged every soul based on its thoughts, words, and deeds in the human world. When the wicked strode the bridge straddling the fiery river, it narrowed to the width of a razor blade (before a demon dragged them into an abyss of woe, where they endured torturous agonies befitting their transgressions). Mercifully, a lovely maiden led virtuous spirits across the bridge and into heaven. Worshipped as a god of truth and integrity by ancient Indo-Iranians (and aligned with Ahura Mazdā in the *Avesta* and Varuṇa in the *Vedas*), Mithra became an important Zoroastrian god due to the vital necessity of honoring oral oaths, in the absence of a writing system, at a time when verbal contracts provided the basic stabilizing force upon which early Iranian civilization thrived.

Mithra therefore embodies an ageless notion of justice, and transgressions of agreements brought swift punishment, for he was regarded as fair—but strict—in their enforcement. His name connotes binding, as in an oath, and Mithra is depicted as having ten thousand eyes to maintain constant vigilance over those who invoke him to seal pacts. During the Last Judgment in Zoroastrianism, at the end of time, Mithra initiates the final sorting of souls according to deed. This event includes a celestial *haoma* (soma) sacrifice that ushers in a restoration of an earthly paradise where death is forever vanquished. [7] For the worthy, eternity is passed in Ahura Mazdā's divine kingdom, in a state of bliss. In this respect, Zoroastrianism contains an idealistic—almost messianic—edge.

As one scholar observes, the prophet Zoroaster first taught the doctrines of individual judgment, heaven and hell, the Last Judgment, and everlasting life in a resurrected body—all of which Judaism, Christianity, and Islam later borrowed. [8] Despite these and other impressive contributions to the history of religion, Zoroaster's own community rejected him and his ideas—a serious hazard of the prophetic occupation (as Muhammad would find out hundreds of years later). However, Zoroaster's exile led to some important early conversions, with a subsequent emphasis on proselytizing, and the rapid diffusion of Zoroastrianism across the Middle East on the heels of its missionaries. As Zoroastrianism developed, proper religious observance grew to mean praying five times a day standing in front of a fire (never to be extinguished); participating in feast days and other festivals following the agricultural calendar (such as New Year celebrations on the spring equinox); adhering to prescribed purity regulations; maintaining good thoughts, words, and deeds; and preserving abundant respect for the natural world. [9]

The daily duties of Zoroastrian priests revolved around the strict recitation of the *Gāthās* every morning, as well as sections of older Avestan scripture. They were also charged with preparing the *yasna* sacrifice, and their focus on rituals involving animals and *haoma* indicate that mystical experiences were evoked through the consumption of plant substances

during sophisticated Zoroastrian rituals designed to alter normal consciousness. Like soma, the exact constitution of the *haoma* formula remains murky: psychoactive mushrooms, cannabis, ephedra, ergot, and
datura are prime candidates for the main ingredients. [10] Without question,
early Iranians knew that most elemental technique of ecstasy—intoxication by hemp. The importance of that understanding is confirmed by the
wide dissemination of the Iranian term for cannabis (*bangha* and its variations) throughout central Asia.

In the *Avesta* scriptures, one finds heroic portrayals of Gustasp and
Ardu who attain wisdom by drinking a hemp elixir, and Zoroaster's wife
Hvovi, who prays for gifts of cannabis potions to strengthen her religious
ardor. [11] Because Zoroaster undertook visionary journeys, aided by cannabis, to commune with the divine, Zoroastrian priests smoked that herb
regularly to induce religious ecstasy. In doing so, they sought to replicate
the inner spiritual experiences of their tradition's founder. [12] As this religion found itself competing with a host of other religious traditions (including Judaism, Manichaeism, and Christianity) between the fourth and
sixth centuries, Zoroastrianism gradually ceded ground to them, and a
hallowed place for cannabis in religious practice continued in the Middle
East.

Religious traditions rarely supersede one another neatly, but instead
tend to overlap as sets of possibilities within a recognizable framework.
For this reason, the veneration of Mithra, Ahura Mazdā, and the goddess
Anahita were not mutually exclusive in the ancient world. [13] Mithra was
worshipped before the rise of Zoroastrianism as a prominent deity of the
sun (and justice) and continued alongside that rival tradition. Much later,
the god Mithra lent his name to a mystery religion (Mithraism) that employed the ritual use of entheogens as a part of spiritual practice—since
they were regarded as providing a regular, reliable, and powerful means
of stimulating alternate states of consciousness (normally the provenance
of the shaman or mystic), which imbue life with new meaning. [14]

At the center of Mithraism was a bull sacrifice (abhorred by Zoroaster). It remains unclear how Mithra worship in pre-Zoroastrian Iran was
transmuted into bull slaying rituals at the heart of the Roman mysteries
centuries later, but depictions of its sacrificial rites are discoverable
across the Middle East and Europe in small Mithraic temples (called
"caves"); the sacrificial aspect of that religion is suggested today in the
Spanish bullfight. As a Roman phenomenon, the Mithraic Mysteries date

from the second century BCE onward. Soldiers, sailors, and imperial officers serving on the empire's frontier provinces, to whom the cult most appealed, participated in ritual purifications, initiatory ordeals, ceremonial meals, and tests of valor before being baptized.

In both his Iranian and Roman iterations, Mithra was associated with the sun, and he took on the role of quasi-savior in escorting the soul through progressive stages of awakening. In Roman Mithraism, initiatory ceremonials ushered aspirants through seven phases of transcendence, which climaxed in a mystical vision of the organizing principles of the universe.[15] During the Eucharist of Mithraism, those present participated in a sacramental feast that contained entheogens. Those sacerdotal meals, sometimes featuring bread and wine (essential symbols in the Christian Eucharist) helped to trigger peak-experiences—and therefore communion in Mithraism was much more than a symbolic reenactment of a sacred myth.

The Mithraic hymns inscribed in Latin beneath the Church of Santa Prisca in Rome demonstrate that ritual practices aimed to bring about salvation or awakening (sometimes described figuratively as rebirth). The following (almost Blakean) lines from the Mithraic liturgy demonstrate that emphasis on the attainment of expanded perception:

Then open your eyes, and you will see the doors open and the world of the gods which is within the doors, so that from the pleasure and joy of the sight your spirit runs ahead and ascends.

So stand still and at once draw breath from the divine into yourself, while you look intently. Then when your soul is restored, say: Come, Lord.[16]

It bears keeping in mind that spiritual restoration required more than the ingestion of plant entheogens; additional components of the Mithraic liturgy included breathing techniques, medicinal recipes, magical rites, charming amulets, and reciting magical words that were at times onomatopoetic, symbolic, or glossolalic (spoken in tongues). All these techniques worked together to usher initiates through several stages to the highest good.[17]

The moment of the bull's sacrifice was highly charged with meaning, since the slain creature was transmuted into a representation of fertility and abundance. In depictions of the ritual slaying, grain springs from the dying bull's tail and sometimes its wounds, features that connect the sacrificial act to ancient fertility rites and notions of rebirth grounded in the changing of the seasons. Practiced widely in the Roman imperial court, including by some emperors, and even a powerful rival to Christianity, Mithraism continued successfully until the conversion of Constantine in 312.[18]

The unexpected rise of Islam in the seventh century resulted in the extinction of Zoroastrian fires that had burned uninterruptedly for hundreds of years, but since insurgent religions often coopted the rituals, texts, or symbols of belief systems that they sought to eclipse or absorb, certain aspects of Zoroastrianism lived on in the new religion (such as ritual prayer five times a day)—as did elements of the Mithraic Eucharist in Christianity. The use of cannabis as part of spiritual observation persisted most conspicuously in the Persian Sufi sects of Islam. To understand the origin of their beliefs, we move to the Arabian Peninsula where seminomadic tribes, though small in number and scattered across the land, traversed a vast desert region.

Although expatriate groups of Zoroastrians, Manichaeans, Mazdakites, and Nestorian Christians immigrated to the Arabian Peninsula prior to the seventh century, and some indigenous tribes flirted with their theologies, the Arabians preferred their own traditional polytheistic belief system. Social cohesion among the Arabian tribes was founded upon unwritten legal codes that validated oral agreements, the worship of a variety of gods (including household and tribal deities), a sacrificial tradition, and a love of poetry.[19] Otherwise, these groups lacked any meaningful centralized organization. For this reason, the stunning rise of those disparate tribes under the banner of a single God took the Byzantine and Persian empires, two global powers of the day, completely by surprise. When the military powerhouse that the prophet Muhammad fashioned thundered onto the world stage following his death, it changed the contours of human civilization within a few hundred years.

Born in the city of Mecca during the mid-sixth century and raised by his uncle (a member of the Quraysh tribe) following the premature death of his parents, Muhammad entered adulthood as a man who although illiterate was well-regarded for his integrity and honor. Always a religiously minded fellow, when his duties as a trader and merchant permitted, Muhammad retreated to nearby caves to practice meditation for weeks at a time. During contemplative sessions in those grottoes, he began to receive revelations through the angel Gabriel, who dictated the Quran to him over two decades. A few years after his first revelation, Muhammad

began to preach an uncompromising form of monotheism grounded firmly in the Judeo-Christian prophetic tradition, and perhaps for this reason,
he initially met with substantial resistance to his proselytizing.

The bold claim that there was only one God, combined with the assertion that Muhammad was his messenger, struck many Meccans as the
height of folly. Muhammad nevertheless gained converts to his new religion, and he insisted on their complete surrender to God (Allah). As he
became a threat to the status quo, opposition to his teachings grew to the
point where it was dangerous for him to remain in the city of his birth. In
622, he abandoned Mecca for the city known today as Medina. Thus
made safe from his enemies, he toiled to convert more people from
polytheism and to unify tribal factions in Medina under his control. Years
later, when Muhammad returned to Mecca with an army of ten thousand
conscripts, he met little resistance to either his message or his leadership.
In the wake of that victory, he destroyed all of the "pagan" shrines and
temples in the city—and then dispatched soldiers across Arabia to do the
same.

When the Eastern Roman emperor Heraclius began to retake portions
of his empire lost to the Iranian Sasanians, Muhammad saw an opportunity to attack when Heraclius struck the Persians (whom the Arab hero
considered heathens). Just two months after consecrating the Ka'aba in
the spring of 632, Muhammad called for war against the Roman Empire. [20] Although the Prophet died shortly thereafter, he successfully converted most of the Arabian Peninsula under the flag of Islam and created
an *ummah* (community or nation) that shared a set of religious and cultural beliefs transmitted in a single language: Arabic. This "commonwealth
of adherents" pledged to follow what we now call the Five Pillars of
Islam: to acknowledge one God and Muhammad as his prophet; to practice ritual prayer five times a day; to contribute funds to charity in accordance with one's station and income; to fast during the holy month of
Ramadan; and to make a pilgrimage to Mecca at least once during one's
lifetime (if at all possible).

Because Mecca was won in battle, the notion of jihad (striving or great
effort) took on dual meanings, and today the term has both outward and
inward dimensions. In its outward form, it sanctions war against the
enemies of Islam. Efforts to vanquish its adversaries grew naturally out of
Muhammad's practice of "holy" warfare, and that martial spirit featured
prominently in early Islamic history and led to the conquest of the entire

Near East. Impressively, Muhammad unified all of Arabia in just ten years—but astonishingly his armies continued onward to challenge Byzantine rule in such distant places as Syria in 636, Iraq in 637, Northern Mesopotamia around 640, Jerusalem and Alexandria in 642, and on it went.[21] To the victorious marauders went the spoils of war, including the horded wealth of Byzantine churches and extensive parcels of land.

Successful martial exploits such as these led to a policy of expansionism that justified the Islamic invasion of vast swathes of the Middle East, Central Asia, and Northern Africa; by the eighth century, Islamic armies made forays into Eastern Europe and Spain. Muslims interpreted the rapid expansion of their empire of faith as definitive proof of God's favor. In truth, its initial successes owed much to the custom of granting substantial autonomy to conquered territories, and sometimes conceding to the exercise of laissez-faire rule. In our own time, this outward manifestation of jihad as justified warfare has been hijacked by violent fringe groups that get lumped together under terms such as "Islamic terrorism." Using the Quran, the Sunnah (the sayings of Muhammad compiled after his death), the Hadith (a proscribed way of life), and the Sharia legal system to justify intolerant beliefs and violent practices, groups such as Al Qaeda and, more recently, the Islamic State of Iraq and Syria (ISIS) have obscured the many cultural achievements of the Muslim religion, and its traditions of tolerance, love, and self-surrender.

In turning to the emergence of Sufism, a form of Islamic mysticism emphasizing a personal quest for direct experience of the divine in the here and now—and not in the afterworld—we recover the inner meaning of jihad as a form of spiritual discipline. Broadly speaking, Sufis seek to overcome their lower (egoic) selves by proceeding through several stages of spiritual development under the guidance of a master teacher (sheikh) to whom obedience is sworn. Sufi aspirants pursue self-annihilation as part of that quest. While strictly speaking there can be no Sufis before the arrival of Islam, the syncretic nature of Sufism brought together contributions from pre-Islamic asceticism, Zoroastrianism, Mithra worship, monastic Christianity, and Neoplatonism to create an enduring Muslim mystical tradition that emphasizes love and ecstatic communion with God.[22]

One way that early Sufi sects in the seventh century established a shared identity was through the coarse woolen clothing that they wore to symbolize their renunciate status. These mystics reveled in finding hidden meanings in the Quran that affirmed their understanding of the inward spiritual development of the Prophet—for such hermeneutical endeavors provided them with touchstones for their own spiritual development. Islamic mystics cite Ḥasan al-Baṣr as an early proponent of the asceticism associated with the Sufi sect. After participating in the early Islamic conquests of Iran, Ḥasan al-Baṣr underwent a change of heart that led him inward. A successful merchant and warrior, Muhammad was active in the world, and therefore Sufis thought that his inward spiritual life sometimes went overlooked by Muslims living more secularly. From the fragments that remain of his sermons, we know that al-Baṣr preached against the dangers of sin, advocated self-examination, and lauded the virtues of an austere way of life. The Sufi propensity for self-denial and the cultivation of religious ecstasy remain uncharacteristic of practices found in mainstream Islam (as codified in the Five Pillars).

An injunction against intoxicants in the Quran means that most Muslims eschew alcohol, but cannabis falls into a nebulous area where it is socially accepted by many Islamic groups, but disdained or prohibited by others. Even so, the use of marijuana for medicinal, religious, aesthetic, and social purposes is well documented in the Islamic world. As an old Arabic proverb provocatively recommends: "If you want to find God, look in a hookah." Abū Yazīd al-Bisṭāmī championed a form of "intoxicated" Islam that drew upon such proverbial wisdom. An ascetic whose grandfather converted to Islam from Zoroastrianism, al-Bisṭāmī emphasized achieving "self-annihilation" (fanā) in the quest for union with God.[23] He experienced intense feelings of "intoxication" in the love of Allah, which led to the death of his egoic self. Borrowing symbolic themes from the Persian court poetry that preceded Islamic literature, he created metaphors of being "drunk" in God, and thereby opened the way for an enduring admixture of ascetic practices and psychoactive intoxicants as a means of achieving ecstatic states of consciousness.

Al-Bisṭāmī turned the Quranic story of the Prophet's night journey to heaven into a trope for the Sufi search for God, and subsequent Sufi mystics adopted that literary device as well. They described their intense longing for God as a state of agony, comparing it to that which a lover feels for an absent beloved. Such estrangement mirrored that which Adam and Eve experienced after the fall as a consequence of bifurcated consciousness. Sufis, however, regard the separation from God as an illusory state of mind resulting from misidentifying the self as the thought stream of the ego. Jalāl al-Dīn Rūmī and other Sufi poets developed extended metaphors of separation and reunion to highlight this point.

Intoxicated Sufis, such as al-Bisṭāmī, attained divine perception through the repetitive recitation of prayer formulas, the continual remembrance of God, energetic dancing and whirling, and playing or listening to religious music. Reportedly, al-Bisṭāmī frequently fainted after issuing the call to prayer, and he would sometimes fall into rapture and utter "blasphemies" such as "Praise be to Me, how great is My Majesty."[24] He claimed to have reached seventy years of age before his mind was fully purified of selfhoods veiling the direct perception of God. When asked his age, he would report it in the number of years following that epiphanic experience—instead of the birthdate of his body.

Similarly, after scrupulously memorizing the Quran in the late ninth and early tenth centuries, one native of Fars, Al-Ḥallāj, sought to uncover hidden meanings in scripture. In that pursuit, his egoic dissolution in the love of God became so profound that he was known to dance in public while declaring: "I am Divine Truth!"[25] Pronouncements such as these struck many orthodox devotees as the pinnacle of hubris, and they were derided as anti-Islamic. For his ecstatic bliss in the love of God, al-Ḥallāj was tortured and killed before public witnesses (following an extended trial marked by indecision and acrimony). So boundless was his love for, and identification with, the Lord that legend recounts him begging forgiveness *of his persecutors and executioners* before his death.

Intensive prayer sessions, dancing to religious orchestrations, reciting mystical poetry, and consuming profuse amounts of cannabis operated synergistically to clarify perception and induce mystical experiences. As one might imagine, wild displays of seemingly irreverent behavior gave rise to rumors of debauchery among some Sufi sects (including charges of pederasty and accusations of hashish-induced malaise). Such disparagements led some "sober" Sufis, along with more orthodox Muslims, to denounce Sufi religious practices and exaggerate the vices of its adherents. Yet, even in the face of continued persecution, their emphasis on love, intoxication, and self-annihilation became inextricably woven into the fabric of Sufi poetry and literature.

Before turning to the two rock stars of Sufi love poetry, Jalāl al-Dīn Rūmī and Mehmed bin Süleyman Fuzuli, we should explicate the trope of the stages (or "stations") a seeker passes through on the way to God. The eleventh-century writer Abu 'Abd al-Rahman al-Sulami belonged to a group of Muslim mystics known as Malāmatiyya. In *Stations of the Righteous*, al-Sulami identifies dozens of waypoints marking progress along the spiritual path. After praising God and emphasizing the need for comportment and discipline to achieve inner repose, even in the midst of strife and tribulation, he notes that the first "station" involves intuitive recognition of the importance of avoiding ostentatious piety, self-conceit, and spiritual pretentions—all of which suggest the continuing machinations of the ego.

As the Sufi seeker progresses further along the inward journey, the stations denote subtle states of perception that he learns to discern from passing thoughts and self-deceptions. The latter stages of spiritual development lead the sincere inquirer to a direct perception of reality, purified of egoic delusion and marked by entrance onto the field of union with God. For al-Sulami, this progression culminated in a revelatory disclosure of secret knowledge concerning the workings of destiny. With the attainment of a state of beatitude untainted by any fear whatsoever, the inward Sufi journey comes to an end.[26] Like the Zen monk who after his enlightenment returns to the marketplace to assist in the salvation of the benighted, the Sufi saint reenters the community unobtrusively to point the way to earnest aspirants embarking on their own journeys to God. The famed poet Farīd ud-Dīn 'Aṭṭār based his celebrated work *Conference of the Birds* on a similar spiritual typography.

In his *Book on the Humble Submission of Those Aspiring*, al-Sulamī warns against the dangers of self-exultation and pride in poverty, and he lauds the virtues of contentment, submission, and inward humility. He explains that the earnest seeker foregoes delusory thought patterns by depriving them of attention. Once that hard-earned accomplishment is in place, the inquirer ceases to expect anything from anyone, and naturally places the interests of others before himself. As he progresses further, the seeker remains humble in public as honors are bestowed on him, and he refuses to accumulate wealth, return to old habits, or to parlay spiritual understanding into a means of gaining recognition.[27] By learning to empty himself of all desire, he turns away from worldly attachments. Only in this way, suggests al-Sulamī, will the Sufi aspirant attain a vision of true reality—an exceedingly arduous task (since it was believed to duplicate the highest spiritual state of the Prophet and his saints).

As a result of the profound nature of that spiritual mission, Sufis count many distinguished intellectuals, writers, and artists among their ranks;

some of them contributed significantly to Islamic spirituality and learning, including Mahmūd Shabistarī (*The Secret Rose Garden*), 'Abd al-Qādir al-Jīlān (*Revelations of the Unseen*), Al-Ghazālī (*The Alchemy of Happiness*), Ibn Sīnā (*The Canon of Medicine*), Mehmed bin Süleyman Fuzuli (*Layla and Majnun*), and the poet-mystic Jalāl al-Dīn Rūmī (*Masnavī*). Many of these notable people learned from the Sufis to disregard the world and its opinions, and to focus instead on inner jihad and the attainment of a realization of God's immanence in the world.

Writers such as Al-Ghazālī rose to defend controversial Sufi religious practices (including dancing and the ritual ingestion of cannabis) against attack from the more orthodox forces that would see them abolished as blasphemies. For instance, in *The Alchemy of Happiness* he contends:

> The heart of man has been so constituted by the Almighty that, like a flint, it contains a hidden fire which is evoked by music and harmony, and renders man beside himself with ecstasy. These harmonies are echoes of that higher world of beauty which we call the world of spirits; they remind man of his relationship to that world, and produce in him an emotion so deep and strange that he himself is powerless to explain it. The effect of music and dancing is deeper in proportion as the natures on which they act are simple and prone to motion; they fan into a flame whatever love is already dormant in the heart, whether it be earthly and sensual, or divine and spiritual.[28]

Al-Ghazālī claims that the Quranic directive to love Allah cannot simply imply obedience to religious law—for that would be tantamount to conformity and a capitulation to commandment over direct religious experience. Rather than unreflectively accepting the moral mandates of orthodox Muslims, Sufis reject the notion that their religiously inspired music and dancing arouses base desires, as some charge—countering that they help to "stir up in themselves greater love towards God."[29] Through musical transport, dedicated Sufi practitioners achieve "spiritual visions and ecstasies, their heart becoming in this condition as clean as silver in the flame of a furnace," and they discover "a degree of purity which could never be attained by any amount of mere outward austerities."[30] In lines such as these, we recognize the language of spiritual alchemy as well.

In his exculpation of the "erotic poetry" read at Sufi gatherings, Al-Ghazālī warns those with shallow spiritual insight from disparaging the ecstasies experienced by the Sufis. "A wise man, though he himself may have no experience of those states," Al-Ghazālī writes, will not deny the "reality of a thing merely because he himself has not experienced it!"[31] His exhortation may serve as a reminder to modern users of cannabis who rarely, if ever, glimpse the divine under its subtle guidance and who remain skeptical concerning claims about it as an entheogen. Asserting a similar point to a twentieth-century audience in regard to the use of psychoactive substances for spiritual purposes, one eloquent scholar of religion, Alan Watts, argues:

> Despite the widespread and undiscriminating prejudice against drugs as such, and despite the claims of certain religious disciplines to be the sole means to genuine mystical insight, I can find no essential difference between the experiences induced, under favorable conditions, by these chemicals and the states of "cosmic consciousness" recorded by R. M. Bucke, William James, Evelyn Underhill, Raynor Johnson, and other investigators of mysticism.[32]

In relation to Al-Ghazālī's defense of intoxicated Islam, and controversial Sufi practices more generally, Watts grasps the fact that authentic peak-experiences are uncorrupted by the chemical agents (or ritual practices) that might serve as their vehicle.

Whether spontaneously occurring, stimulated by "taking a pill or chewing a plant," or generated through religious practice, peak-experiences offer the possibility of a new way of being—one that "can be matured and deepened by the various ways of meditation in which drugs are no longer necessary or useful." Authentic transcendental experiences enable an "individual to be so peculiarly open and sensitive to organic reality that the ego begins to be seen for the transparent abstraction that it is."[33] The importance of such miraculous openings to otherwise unrecognized states of consciousness are not diminished by their fleeting nature; these foretastes of a different quality of mind point toward a reality always with us, but too often unrecognized. Peak-experiences, which represent an important response to the panhuman yearning for paradise, must be deepened through spiritual practices such as meditation to bring presence, mindfulness, or emptiness more permanently to the fore of consciousness. As one learns to live more in stillness by dissolving the egoic thought-stream in the light of attention, one increasingly meets with forceful feelings of peacefulness, blessedness, and a sense of melting into the totality that characterize full and sustained awakening.

The Sufi insistence on making cannabis part of spiritual practice is attributable to the fact that, in the right-minded person, marijuana facilitates a heightened state of concentration that can deepen contemplation. For Sufis ascribing to the "intoxication" school, hashish is a holy sacrament that stimulates mild feelings of euphoria and lends acquiescence and carefreeness. It bestows feelings of jocularity and amiability.[34] These same qualities made the plant popular among Sufis living communally, and they helped to guarantee a space for the creative expression of their musicians, dancers, poets, and artists. Perhaps one measure of the enduring influence of Sufi practices on the Islamic world are the throngs of Muslims who still use preparations of cannabis (as bhang, ganja, or hashish) for a variety of purposes in Iran, Afghanistan, Pakistan, India, and kif (alternately spelled "kef," "kief," or "keef") in North Africa—despite prohibitions against intoxicants in the Sharia.

A cannabis culture persists in parts of the Islamic Middle East in the form of a covert "green language" in popular lore. Cannabis is green, the color of Islam,[35] and also of the so-called hidden prophet of Sufism, *al-Khiḍr* or the *Green Man*—a vegetative spirit traditionally associated with fecundity, but later with the Sufi sect more generally.[36] Apocryphally, Sheik Qutb ad-Dīn Haydar, the founder of a movement of dervishes in Iran, discovered the spiritual applications of marijuana and passed that knowledge on to his followers.[37] Orthodox Muslims, who considered Sufis radical outlaws, referred pejoratively to them as *hashishiyya* (hashish users or even assassins).[38] In fact, cannabis became so integral to religious communal life among Sufi sects that outsiders often thought them dissidents and subversives. Nevertheless, their herb of choice continued to be celebrated in Islamic poetry, where it was conflated with the "wine of paradise" in the Quran and gave rise to a proliferation of metaphors of intoxication with God as their referent.

Sufis justified their nonconformist religious pursuits by grounding them in nuanced interpretations of the Quran. In reading beyond literal levels of meaning in Quranic *surahs* (chapters), they claimed to eliminate the veil that obscures ultimate reality (*ḥaqīqah*) from ordinary perception. Over time, the Sufis developed ways of glossing other parts of the canon, too. They sought out (and found) esoteric meanings believed intelligible only to those who had reached certain levels of spiritual understanding. In his treatise "On the Divine Essence," the eighteenth-century Sufi Ahmad ibn ʿAjiba followed the celebrated mystic philosopher ibn al-ʿArabī in referencing "a subtle, luminous, radiant, spiritual structure without corporeality" that can be described only by resorting to negative expressions, for it has no form, no limitation, no substance, and no body. God is "the Necessary Being who reveals Himself through every existing thing!"[39]

When one has drunk from the "Eternal Wine," claims ibn 'Ajiba, that resplendent Essence reveals itself to the eye of the heart through all material forms. He locates scriptural testimony to this unity "in the words of the Prophet: 'God was, and nothing was with Him.'" That is to say, "in eternity, there is neither form nor delimitation, nor sensory aspect, nor category."[40] As such, that which appears in the phenomenal world already participates completely and wholly in the eternal. When a Sufi attains that heightened state of perception, oppositions between the inner and outer—self and other—disintegrate. This eradication of duality marks the apex of the Islamic Sufi "vision quest," for through it, what was once hidden is made manifest.

In part due to the many translations of his monumental work *Māsnavī* (composed of more than twenty thousand rhymed couplets), the Persian poet Jalāl al-Dīn Rūmī remains the most renowned Sufi in the West. In his book, the illusory state of separation from God felt by the unenlightened seeker becomes a central conceit. Rūmī compares the yearning of the aspirant for the divine to that of a lover for the beloved, but most famously to a reed-like plant ripped from the riverbed. Extending the latter metaphor, he figuratively transforms the severed reed into a flute whose plaintive song evokes that painful estrangement:

> Now listen to this reed-flute's deep lament
> About the heartache being apart has meant:
> "Since from the reed-bed they uprooted me
> My song's expressed each human agony
> A breast which separation's split in two
> Is what I seek, to share this pain with you
> When kept from their true origin, all yearn
> For union on the day they can return."[41]

In these lines, "return" does not refer to the death of the body only, although physical dissolution in the eternal may be part of the intended meaning. What is asserted in the figurative poetic language of the text is a return to a state of unified perception. The songs of the reed (i.e., Rūmī's couplets) contain deep secrets, but many "eyes and ears can't penetrate the veil" and see that body and soul are already "joined to form one whole."[42] Until that ego-imposed separation is banished, the reed flute will sing and open willing hearts to the truth of God's oneness—a theme that runs like a steady stream through the writings of the Sufis.

The inquisitive reader anxious to extend this brief foray into Islamic literatures of intoxication beyond the Sufis should take heart that there was hardly an Arabic poet between the thirteenth and sixteenth centuries who did not refer to cannabis.[43] Even today, the sweetmeat majoun (ma'jun) made from marijuana leaves mixed with flour, milk, butter, and sugar, is sold in marketplaces throughout India and the Middle East. It may also be prepared as a medicinal confection. So entrenched is the use of cannabis in modern Arabic culture that the sober poet Nizār Qabbānī bemoaned that in a land of prophets, when the moon rises in the East, "people leave their shops and walk in groups / To meet the moon / Carrying bread, hashish, and phonographs to the mountain tops."[44]

Indeed, hashish ingestion became exceptionally popular from the early twelfth century onward in the Middle East, and a "clandestine" literary life of that plant can be traced through the literatures of the region. The widely read collection of stories *1,001 Nights*, for instance, satirically describes hashish's aphrodisiac properties in the "Tale of the Hashish Eater," "The Tale of Two Hashish Eaters," and "Tale of the Second Captain of Police." In a thirteenth-century poem on the ever-popular topic of hashish and wine, the poet Al-Isʻirdī imagines an animated contest between the two substances in which the virtues of "the green one" become readily apparent:

You have asked about the relationship between the green one and wine. Thus listen to
What a person of correct and straightforward views has to say.

Surely wine does not possess some of the qualities of hashish.
Can it be drunk openly in a Sufi monastery or a mosque?

You ought to obtain it, a green one, not to be acquired at an excessive price
For the white of silver or the red of gold.

Rather, in contrast to wine, it comes as a gift
Removed from purchase without the need for abstemiousness.

It is something belonging to meadows whose greenness resembles the gardens of Paradise,
Whereas their wine is like a burning firebrand.

Their wine makes you forget all the meanings there are, while this one
Recalls the secrets of Beauty declared unique.

It is the secret. In it, the spirit ascends to the highest
Spots on a heavenly ascent of disembodied understanding.

Rather it is, indeed, the spirit itself.[45]

In addition to asserting that cannabis augments spiritual perception, this
passage illustrates the "green language" employed by Islamic poets. It
also emphasizes some of the properties that endeared that herb to Sufis,
poets, and laypersons. As the fourteenth-century writer Ṣafī al-Dīn al-Ḥill
maintained: "Hashish makes you dispense with wine, / The new leaves
with the old one, / And the green one with pure red wine. How great is the
difference between emerald and carnelian!" The poet argues that hashish
inflicts on the partaker "no hangover, except subtle thinking / That cheers
the soul to the last breath. An intoxication such as that wine is unable to
offer."[46]

In a similar vein, the sixteenth-century Ottoman poet Fuzuli belonged
to an elite group of Sufis who found hashish to be a master teacher. In
Beng ü Bâde (*Hashish and Wine*), he recognizes the unfolding of mystic
love as the highest purpose of the religious quest. For that reason, Fuzuli
concludes that a sheik of love finds refuge in cannabis (whereas wine
may only point the way to that truth), and he defends the potential for
cannabis to contribute to overall self-betterment.[47] In his poem *Bangāb-
nāma* (*Book of the Pothead*), Maḥmūd Baḥrī, a seventeenth-century Muslim Allen Ginsberg, eulogizes the cannabis beverage bhang (*bhangab*)
and advises his readers thusly:

> Drink your *bhangab* and be happy—
> Be a dervish and put your heart at peace.
> Lose all your life in drinking this exhilaration,
> And not in sewing shabby clothes.[48]

Later in life, when Baḥrī became a mystic recluse independent of any
sectarian affiliation, his poetry continued to draw upon an established
tradition of Sufi lyricism—only he went a step further than other "intoxicated" poets by leaving little doubt that his references to bhang had literal, as well as allegorical, meanings.[49]

While the proposition of following further literary references to cannabis in the Islamic tradition is tempting, let us continue onward and
explore the medical and spiritual uses of cannabis in (and around) China.

In doing so, we shift from an emphasis on the consciousness raising potential of cannabis to its role in the traditional pharmacopeia of indigenous cultures. In anticipation of that discussion, we presuppose an integral relationship between the mind and the body, one that may be tapped to enhance the efficacy of other modalities of healing. As the Zen luminary Shunryu Suzuki reminds us, the body and mind are "not two, and not one."[50]

3

CHINESE PHARMACOPOEIA AND THE GOLDEN FLOWER

Chinese civilization is the oldest in continuous existence, and hemp cultivation in that region of the world dates back millennia. From approximately 10000 BCE onward, central and eastern Asian peoples began to rely on hemp to make rope, fish netting, canvas, and fabrics—and it became a staple source of food for the Han Chinese and their animals. The seeds of the hemp plant provided a life-nourishing combination of protein and essential fatty acids, as well as important minerals like magnesium, calcium, and potassium.[1] Proper preparation made hemp seeds more easily digestible, and they contained very little tetrahydrocannabinol (THC) when hulled and cleaned.

Some of the earliest references to hemp and its role in traditional agrarian life appear in founding documents of Chinese culture, such as the *Book of Songs* (*Shijing*), *Bamboo Annals* (*Zhushu Jinian*), and the *Book of Rites* (*Liji*). The oldest lyrical poems in the *Book of Songs* date to around 1100 BCE (though they were collated and anthologized five hundred years later). During that formative period, rival feudal states led by powerful warlords regularly fought one another for supremacy—much to the detriment of the common people who scratched a meager existence out of the land. Two of the most powerful kingdoms, the Shang (c. 1700–1000 BCE) and succeeding Zhou (c. 1000–250 BCE), gave their names to dynasties that preceded the formal unification of China under the imperial rule of Emperor Qin Shi Huang (in the second century BCE).

The *Book of Songs* offers an idealized portrait of Zhou society with such effortless grace that it earned a place among the *Five Classics* of the traditional Confucian canon.[2] The first Chinese person to dedicate his life to teaching, the sage Confucius (Kongzi) placed considerable emphasis on studying the *Book of Songs*, and he reinterpreted that text to make it conform to codes of propriety, which he formulated to create a more harmonious society. In doing so, he reimagined life during the late Shang and early Zhou dynasties as an idyllic model for peaceful coexistence—a vision that he offered as a foil to the war-filled Spring and Autumn Period (770–476 BCE) into which the great educator was born.

This backward glance implicit in the Confucian celebration of Zhou culture (as depicted in the *Book of Songs*) helped to shape the contours of Chinese civilization for centuries by providing an alternate vision of human nature as good, while grounding cultural traditions firmly in the past. In accord with his belief in human perfectibility, Confucius advocated lifelong learning, extolled the virtues of literature and art, and dreamt of social betterment resulting from leadership by persons of superior virtue. In addition, he outlined a hierarchy of relationships for all members of society centered on the "golden rule" of altruism and conscientiousness: to "not do to others what you do not want them to do to you."[3]

The *Book of Songs* includes folk tunes, songs of the nobility, ritual hymns, and lyrical ballads addressing topics ranging from ancestor worship, the concerns of commoners, to the affairs of members belonging to the ruling house.[4] Together, these poems create a complex (though not always coherent) account of life in the various kingdoms of the late Shang and early Zhou periods—though of the more than three hundred poems that make up the *Book of Songs*, just five are attributable to the preceding Shang dynasty.[5] The archaic simplicity of many of them evokes a pastoral "golden age" when individuals lived harmoniously with each other and with nature.

Due to the centrality of hemp to everyday life during the Shang and Zhou dynasties, many poems in the *Book of Songs* reference cannabis. In one such work, the marriage customs in the Lu and Qi kingdoms (in modern Shangdong province) are highlighted, and the process of negotiating a nuptial agreement is compared to planting cannabis. The absence of affectation in songs such as this one recalls the pastoral innocence that Confucius found so worthy of emulation:

> Over the southern hill so deep

> The male fox drags along,
> But the way to Lu is easy and broad
> For this Qi lady on her wedding-way.
> Yet once she has made the journey,
> Never again must her fancy roam.
>
> Fiber shoes, five pairs;
> Cap ribbons, a couple.
> The way to Lu is easy and broad
> For this lady of Qi to use.
> But once she has used it,
> No way else must she ever go.
>
> When we plant hemp, how do we do it?
> Across and along we put the rows.
> When one takes a wife, how is it done?
> The man must talk with her father and mother.
> And once he has talked with them,
> No one else must he court.[6]

In undertaking the journey to her husband's house in the kingdom of Lu (carrying her dowry gifts), this maiden of Qi must leave behind her home, her family, and her childhood. In return, her husband relinquishes all intimate ties with other women.

The hemp poems in the *Book of Songs* were sometimes sung a cappella or with light musical accompaniment, such as in this celebration of the fecundity of the kingdom of Liu:

> Among the hillocks grows the hemp;
> There works Zi-jue of Liu
> There works Zi-jue of Liu
> If only he would come in and rest!
>
> Among the hillocks grows the wheat;
> There works Zi-guo of Liu,
> There works Zi-guo of Liu,
> If only he would come in to supper!
>
> Among the hillocks grow the plum trees;
> There work those good men of Liu,
> There work those good men of Liu,
> That gave me jet-stones for my girdle.

The lyrical placement of hemp along with wheat (a staple food) and plum trees (from which delicious wines are made) makes evident the prominence of hemp in ancient Chinese culture.

One final selection from a song cycle provides a literary illustration of the close-knit community that Shang and Zhou peasants forged—bound as they were to collective agricultural duties (such as sowing and reaping fields) during the summer and fall months. Although filled with toil, their lives were sustained by the natural abundance brought forth regularly during the year. One can imagine the song in unison celebrating those harvests:

> In the sixth month we eat wild plums and cherries,
> In the seventh month we boil mallows and beans.
> In the eighth month we dry the dates,
> In the tenth month we take the rice
> To make it with the spring wine,
> So that we may be granted long life.
> In the seventh month we eat the melons,
> In the eighth month we cut the gourds,
> In the ninth month we take the seeding hemp,
> We gather bitter herbs, we cut the ailanthus for firewood,
> That our husbandman may eat. [7]

Here, seed-laden hemp plants are cultivated alongside other "bitter herbs" used in the manufacture of medications (as an old Chinese proverb has it: "good medicine tastes bitter" 良药苦口). This juxtaposition of cannabis-medicine with an emphasis on the importance of eating a variety of healthy foods speaks to the holistic approach to human health adopted by practitioners of traditional Chinese medicine.

Perhaps surprisingly, given the importance of hemp in Chinese culture as a food grain (as well as an important source of oil and raw fiber for building), cannabis was not generally cultivated for its psychoactive properties. As a medicine, however, evidence exists of cannabis flowers and leaves being utilized in the Middle Kingdom as early as the third millennium BCE. [8] Yet, that plant's manifold medicinal attributes earned it a only a modest place in Chinese pharmacopoeia, where it was deployed like any healing herb—within the context of a highly complex understanding of human physiology and the natural world that we generally refer to as "Traditional Chinese Medicine" in the West.

Traditional Chinese Medicine emerged from an admixture of various indigenous shamanistic healing arts (from the pre-Confucian era) and Ayurvedic medicine from India. Following the introduction of important Indian medical principles, the Chinese tradition of healing developed independently—for astronomy, arithmetic, agronomy, and medicine were always traditional areas of inquiry in the Middle Kingdom.[9] In fact, the relationship between religious practice and medicine in China predated the arrival of Indian Buddhism (in shamanism and religious Daoism), and the existence of a body-mind-spirit continuum is a defining feature of Eastern medicine more generally.

Cannabis first appears in the *Classic of Herbal Medicine* (*Shen Nong Bencaojing*). Attributed by name to Emperor Shen Nong, but most likely compiled during the first or second century BCE, it remains a seminal text in the branch of Chinese medicine dealing with herbs and herbal remedies. It catalogs medications derived from plant, animal, and mineral products deployed to invigorate and prolong life, prevent illness, and therapeutically treat disease. In the entry for cannabis sativa, known in Chinese as *dama* (大麻), the resinous flowers of the plant are described as sweet, balanced, and best suited to treat "seven damages" (including the exhaustion of energy and a weak pulse), as well as problems associated with the five *zang* organs (or viscera).[10]

While the protracted use of cannabis enabled one "to communicate with the spirit light" and made the body buoyant, excessive dosages might cause one to see ghosts or "frantically run about"! Even so, the seeds of the cannabis plant were recognized as an energy (qi) boost, and the *Classic of Herbal Medicine* assured readers concerned with the long-term effects of cannabis that it "may make one fat" and strong, but never senile. In acknowledgment of their oft-reported aphrodisiac effects, or perhaps their elongated shape, the *Classic of Herbal Medicine* refers to cannabis flowers as *ma bo* (麻勃, or hemp erection).[11]

Once urged by a legendary emperor to farm mulberry trees (in support of silk worm production) and to cultivate hemp, the Chinese people learned to use every part of the cannabis plant medicinally: male flowers for menstrual disorders and wounds, the oil for hair loss and throat dryness, the stalk as a diuretic and to dislodge urinary tract stones, and the juice of the root to expel a retained placenta. The leaves were made into an extract to rid the body of intestinal parasites; hemp seeds, applied topically, were reputed to clear heat from sores and ulcerations.[12] Although traditionally regarded as a subdivision of the mulberry family, modern taxonomy tends to place cannabis in the Cannabaceae family of small flowering plants, with its closest relative being hops (a basic ingredient in beer). [13]

Since they did not appeal directly to the Han psyche as much as alcohol, the psychoactive effects of cannabis generally received scant attention from practitioners of traditional Chinese medicine. One prominent exception was the renowned third-century physician Hua Tuo (c. 140–208) who in addition to practicing moxibustion and acupuncture—two important Chinese treatment modalities—employed a wine and cannabis powder preparation as an anesthetic for the abdominal and gastrointestinal surgical procedures that he was innovating. Such invention suggests that some of Hua Tuo's approaches to medicine have roots in the Hindu Ayurvedic system of medicine.

Hua Tuo's experiments with cannabis and surgery came to a tragic end when he was executed, and his writings burned, for failing to serve promptly at the whim of Emperor Cao Cao. That single ignorant decision by the emperor set back the advancement of medical science in China by hundreds of years. However, Cao Cao lived to regret slaying Hua Tuo, for he suffered debilitating headaches (and Hua Tuo alleviated his throbbing cranial pain, but could not resolve the underlying condition without surgery). If such anguish were not evidence enough of karmic justice, one of Cao Cao's favored sons died at the age of twelve for lack of a doctor with the talents of Hua Tuo. Still, much more was lost with the doctor's execution than the life of a young princeling, for the art of surgery that Hua Tuo was revolutionizing never found a place in Traditional Chinese Medicine again.

During the first and second centuries Indian monks brought considerable medical knowledge with them to China, along with Buddhism, by way of the Silk Road—a network of trade routes that connected the Far East with the West. Healers in both India and China recognized integral relationships among mind, body, and spirit centuries in advance of their counterparts in the West. They envisioned the human organism as inextricably interconnected with the natural world through a web of microcosmic and macrocosmic relationships. Rather than standing outside of an environment that he sought to subjugate, the human being was deemed subject to the same universal forces and patterns that shape other physical phenomena in the universe.

Out of such a vision arose elaborate theories concerning the nature of energy (qi) and how it circulates with the blood through channels (or meridians) in the body—just as water flows through rivers and tributaries on the earth. [14] By inferring patterns from nature and projecting them onto the human body, diseases could be compared, for instance, to flooding resulting from blockages (like silt in rivers). Sickness originated with imbalances that emerged internally or in relationship to external reality. [15] Emotional shifts, improper diet, physical exhaustion, and excessive sexual activity might be internal causes of illness, while abnormal changes in the weather or other encounters with cold, heat, dampness, or dryness could be external sources of disease.

Although the dominant features of Chinese medicine, and the analogic thinking that informs them, elude simple summary, adept practitioners understand that qi springs out of a vital active force without distinction of form or figure, called *li*, which permeates the universe. Qi has a dual nature as yin and yang, the opposite (yet complementary) forces that roughly correspond to positive and negative electrical charges. [16] The eighteenth-century Chinese masterwork *Dream of the Red Chamber* (*Honglou meng*) contains a scene that fittingly illustrates the complementary bipolarity of yin and yang: an elegant young lady, named Xiang-yun, educates a curious maid concerning the manner in which yin and yang forces give to all material things their distinctive forms. Yin and yang, she observes, are manifested in the "10,000 things" of the world (i.e., all material things). The earth is yin, while sky is yang; likewise, water is yin, while fire is yang. Every sentient being contains these complementary forces—as do nonsentient life forms such as trees, plants, flowers, stones, and bricks. Subtler still, in a single leaf of a tree, yin and yang are present. As Xiang-yun explains, "the side facing upwards toward the sky" is yang, while "the underside, facing toward the ground" is yin. [17]

Consequently, yin and yang should not be regarded as static categories, but instead as dynamic processes in a state of unceasing transformation. In the tension between the poles of yin and yang exists the energy that sustains all life: when yin is exhausted, it becomes yang—and the converse is also true. The alternation of day and night provides another example of these cyclic complementary movements, for when the "yang" of the day is spent, it gives rise to the "yin" of the night. The transition between the two is deemed so subtle and gradual that determining precisely where one ends and the other begins becomes impossible (without arbitrary distinctions such as those of mechanical time)—because they are a single process. According to such a worldview, life itself is a dynamic unfolding in which yin forces (static, internal, descending, cold, and dark) alternate with yang forces (dynamic, external, rising, warm, and bright) throughout the cosmos. Their cyclical patterns of alternation mold everything in the world—with each variation in nature being directly attributable to different combinations of those forces.

The transformative potential of yin and yang finds expression in the Five Phases (*Wu Xing*). Collectively, these five principles represent the fundamental qualities and behavioral patterns intrinsic in the cosmos and exist as an unceasing process of transformation. All matter is subject to the five states of molecular vibration, which in turn correspond to the Five Phases that express the inherent propensity for growth in all things (i.e., the natural movement of a germinated seed into a fully grown tree). More nuanced still, each of the Five Phases has a correlate in one of the five elements (wood, earth, fire, metal, and water), which likewise exhibit particular tendencies. Wood stands for a process of germination and a movement of spreading outward, like seeds being sown, while earth represents nourishment and a tendency toward containment. Fire is emblematic of heat and growth with an impulse for flaring upward, metal implies a maturing process and a concentrating influence, and water denotes coolness, decay, transmutation, and downward flow. A broader cyclic pattern is discerned in the movement of the five elements, one that ensures that equilibrium abides among the five, so that one element does not dominate over others and cause imbalance (and subsequently illness): wood loosens earth, fire melts metal, earth obstructs water, metal cuts wood, and water extinguishes fire.[18]

The Five Elements find analogs in the five *zang* organs of the human body: the liver, heart, spleen, lung, and kidneys (wood, fire, earth, metal, and water respectively). In Traditional Chinese Medicine, great importance is placed on understanding the sinuous relationships among the *zang* and *fu* organs, so as to properly identify and treat symptoms of physical and mental illnesses. The six *fu* organs (the large and small intestines, gall bladder, urinary bladder, stomach, and triple-burner "*sanjiao*") work with the five *zang* organs to expedite the secondary functions of absorbing and expelling nutrients. The "*zang-fu*" viscera operate in tandem with a meridian system of interdependent networks (or pathways) along which qi and blood move through the body. When qi flows freely through that network, and yin and yang are balanced, the body is protected from illness.

All told, there are twenty channels in the human body's meridian system—each with unique branches, collaterals, and corresponding acupoints. The acupoint system might be envisioned as overlaid atop the circuits of energy and blood that make up the meridian system. Since the *zang-fu* organs and meridian system promote communication between the human body and the outer world, they are used to discover the cause of disease and formulate proper courses of treatment. Additionally, due to the multifarious ways in which the *zang-fu* organs interact with the meridian system, each organ has multiple functions. The lungs drive respiration, as well as olfactory processes. The heart circulates blood and qi, but it is also the site of the mind (where consciousness and psychological phenomena take place).[19] In both medicine and philosophy, many translators render the term *xin* (心) as "heart-mind" in order to capture its dual nature in Chinese thinking.

In Traditional Chinese Medicine, diagnosis is achieved through visual inspection of the patient's deportment, mental state, facial affect, and tongue. Moreover, attentive listening to the quality of a patient's voice, smelling the breath, and studying the tongue augment a sophisticated technique of pulse taking.[20] In terms of voice reading, low moans indicate kidney problems, heavy sighing points to spleen and intestinal difficulties, choking and crying suggests trouble with the lungs, and verbose irritability may mean heart dysfunction. As to tongue reading, the color of its tip reveals the condition of the heart, its center the stomach and spleen, its edges the liver and gall bladder, while the underside indicates the function of the kidneys.[21]

Diagnostic pulse taking requires great skill and heightened astuteness, as three main pulses must be discerned *in the same spot*—and up to twelve acupoints run from just above the wrist along the radial artery to the elbow. In each of these positions, four degrees (strong, feeble, slow, and hasty) of the three pulses must be distinguished. So integrated are the diagnostic techniques available to the practitioner of Traditional Chinese Medicine that the condition of the ears might reveal something important about the health of the kidneys, just as the eyebrows would concerning the bone marrow. Moreover, once physical or functional imbalances become entrenched in organs, they create receptivity toward certain states of consciousness. Liver stagnation might lead to depression, frustration, or angry outbursts.[22]

Similarly, emotional outpourings might cause a flare up of qi, while feelings of deep sadness weaken it. In either case, they destabilize the natural harmonious stasis of the body. The trained practitioner of Chinese medicine seeks to cure both the minds of her patients and their bodies—a holistic approach to the restoration of health that developed out of the body-mind-spirit continuum. She might counsel patients concerning the essential relationship between consciousness and the physical body by emphasizing the need for proper nourishment, the central role of qi and blood flow in restoring vigor, and the importance of meditation and physical exercise. Traditional Chinese Medicine is therefore simultaneously preventative and curative.

In respect to the prevention of illness, traditional Chinese doctors devote special attention to keeping yin and yang in equilibrium in the body through proper diet. Food is regarded as medicine, and a good meal should include a mixture of tastes and temperatures in the dishes (sweet/ bitter, spicy/mild, hot/cool) so as to match the qualities of the Five Phases.[23] Meals are balanced because the dominant characteristics of every ingredient affects organs differently. If an organ is already out of balance, disrupting the smooth accord of the body and mind, certain foods may exacerbate that disharmony (or conversely help restore it to equilibrium). Physical exercises, such as *qigong, taijiquan*, or meditation, also assist in circulating blood and qi through the body. In modern China, it remains commonplace to see groups of people, often of retirement age, practicing these and other exercises in parks and green spaces across the country.

Although diet and exercise remain important, stronger treatments are generally required to restore the body's innate capacity to self-regulate after a disease process becomes entrenched. In such cases, practitioners of Traditional Chinese Medicine might prescribe a combination of herbal remedies, acupuncture, moxibustion, and cupping to break up blockages and restore the imbalances that cause illness. As a modality of treatment, acupuncture developed over thousands of years in China from various bloodletting practices and techniques of applying heated compresses.[24] Eventually, acupuncture grew into its own discipline employing needles of various lengths and shapes to drain ulcers or sores, and to stimulate the flow of qi through the meridian system of the body.

In total, acupoints in the human body number in the hundreds, and they are found from the top of the head to the bottom of the feet. Because of the intricate nature of the interrelationships between the body and cosmos (only hinted at in this brief overview), the proper needling of acupoints located along the large intestine channel of the hand might ease a distorted face.[25] Moxibustion as a treatment modality involves burning mudwort (moxa) over specific acupoints to draw toxins away from the body. Sometimes Chinese doctors transfer that heat from the body and into small glass cups, which leave round red patches on the skin when removed (but which heal after several days). If cold has penetrated deeply, then heat applied to the proper spot on the body for the correct duration of time has a curative effect by stimulating qi and encouraging healing.

Herbal medications have a long history in China as another means of rectifying imbalances in the body. Chinese doctors practicing herbal medicine mix plant, animal, and mineral ingredients into prescriptions designed to treat patients' unique physical and mental conditions. Some herbal formulations serve as standard prescriptions to treat disease, but such decoctions are regularly customized to suit the particularities of each illness. Every ingredient in an herbal prescription is understood to have significant synergetic ramifications upon the others, which are modulated using a hierarchical theory (of monarch, minister, assistant, and guide) that takes years to learn comprehensively. Basically, each prescription has a key ingredient (the "monarch"), which the "minister" supports, while "assistants" strengthen it, and "guides" direct the medicines to the proper locations in the body.[26]

Therefore, in every Chinese herbal medical prescription, a proper ordering among ingredients must be achieved so that they may work in unison to restore vitality to the body and mind. These hierarchical roles for herbal ingredients mirror those once found in imperial Chinese society, and they are part and parcel of a view of the universe where everything has its proper place (a notion that bears some resemblance to the Great Chain of Being in the West). Critically, the Chinese physician must understand the effects of each prescription ingredient, as well as how it interacts with the other compounds—all within the context of the aforementioned systems of the body. With such a comprehension in place, she develops thoughtful strategies for treatments of her patients' illnesses. Whether her herbal prescriptions are long or short, ingredients must be cleaned, dried, ground, or crushed and made into pastes or herbal pouches for boiling (or storage for later use). They are administered as decoctions, pills, powders, plasters, medical wines, and syrups. [27]

Although traditional Chinese medicine does not generally exploit the psychotropic effects of cannabis in medical prescriptions (since Hua Tuo's recipes for cannabis powder anesthetics were lost), a wide variety of plants with powerful mental and physical effects on the human body remain part of that pharmacopoeia. For example, most traditional sedating formulas feature aconite and datura as primary ingredients. Datura, recognized in many cultures as a strong hallucinogen, was considered an effective spasmolytic, analgesic, anti-asthmatic, and general anesthetic. [28] Likewise, the stems of the Chinese ephedra plant were judged effective in alleviating the symptoms of cough, cold and fever, and fluid retention in the body. [29] Because of the complexity of the body and its channels, the relationships between the inner and the outer worlds, and the synergic interactions between prescription ingredients, only the most skilled physicians gain a comprehensive mastery of plant medicines in the Chinese tradition.

Historically, the knowledge of herbs in China was surrounded in secrecy. Most ancient and medieval shaman-magician-healer-priest practitioners of herbal healing held tightly to their esoteric knowledge, as it ensured them an esteemed place in society. For this reason, the shaman is a key figure in the development of Chinese medicine. When shamanistic medico-religious practices were repressed beginning in the Han dynasty (206 BCE–220 CE) as state authorized religions commanded imperial favor, shamanism merged with religious Daoism as a way to survive. Unlike philosophical Daoism, which we will discuss in more detail below, religious Daoism emphasizes ritualistic, ceremonial, and alchemical exercises in which herbal and mineral brews are quaffed in the quest to achieve immortality (in this life, or in the hereafter). In their alchemical rites, the transmutation of base elements, such as iron into pure gold, symbolically exemplifies the physical and mental transformations that one undergoes on the road to salvation.

In this way, the secret art of medical herbalism in (pre-Daoist) Chinese shamanism preserved an esoteric understanding of enlightenment often obscured by the alchemical language used in the practice of religious Daoism. Religious Daoists who trained in alchemy were well aware of the psychoactive and entheogenic properties of cannabis, and they undoubtedly knew how to manufacture hemp-based incenses and elixirs for ceremonial occasions. Although references to cannabis in Daoist literatures are rare, the custom of burning cannabis to drive away evil ghosts is featured in a sixth-century literary anthology titled *Essentials of the Matchless Books* (*Wu Shang Pi Yao*). One guesses that the smoke from Daoist incense burners had a salutary effect upon people gathered for the ceremonial occasions on which it was burnt. Perhaps another indication of the centrality of cannabis to religious Daoism is the hemp maiden, Ma Gu—one of eight major deities revered by the Daoist sect of the Highest Clarity School on Maoshan Mountain (in modern-day Jiangsu province).[30]

Alchemy, it was noted, symbolizes spiritual transformation in the transmutation of base metals into gold. For that reason, the quest of religious Daoists after the "Elixir of Life" (drinkable gold) was more about gaining transcendence over human mortality than manufacturing longevity for the body—and for such purposes they took mind-enhancing substances as early as the third century BCE.[31] The pills and elixirs of transformation brewed and deemed effectual bestowed upon their makers the status of masters of esoteric compounds, and their herbal medicines were combined with meditation and other exercises to effect spiritual transformation (along with bodily health). Unfortunately, charlatan purveyors of religious Daoism and alchemy inadvertently, but all too frequently, poisoned themselves and others (including some emperors) with elixirs laced with mercury, lead, and sulfur. Those infusions must have been quite beautiful to gaze upon: eternity in a cup. But all too often, they were deadly.

In contrast to the wizards of religious Daoism who studied alchemy to live forever, philosophical Daoists followed the mystical teachings recorded by Laozi in the fourth century BCE. According to legend, Laozi wrote the elegant verses that make up the *Dao de Jing* (*Book of the Way*) at the request of a prescient border guard when the sage passed through a remote frontier post. On the other side of it, Laozi sought a rustic life far from the chaos of warring feudal states. The poems that make up the *Dao de Jing* are largely free of magic, alchemy, or references to herbal medicines, and instead offer lessons on a mode of being through which life is lived naturally, effortlessly, and in harmony with the *dao* (path, way, or principle) that sustains the cosmos.

In the passages below, we gain a better appreciation for the subtlety of the *dao*, as well as the challenge of putting one's mind in accord with it (for it cannot be grasped). Like a well, it is never depleted, and like a void, it is filled only with pure potential. The *dao* remains "hidden but always present," and though it gives birth to all things, it "does not take sides."[32] The ancient Daoist masters were vigilant, present, supple, and they continually set their minds on reality and the actuality of things. Thus these sages discovered a state of consciousness that the reader is asked to attain by emulating their equipoise:

> They were careful
> as someone crossing an iced-over stream.
> Alert as a warrior in enemy territory.
> Courteous as a guest.
> Fluid as melting ice.
> Shapeable as a block of wood.
> Receptive as a valley.
> Clear as a glass of water.
>
> Do you have the patience to wait
> till your mud settles and the water is clear?
> Can you remain unmoving
> till the right action arises by itself?
>
> The Master does not seek fulfillment.
> Not seeking, not expecting,
> she is present, and can welcome all things.[33]

For philosophical Daoists, the aim of life is to live in stillness—free from prejudice, ideology, or desire. Their state of consciousness is not one of passive resignation, but rather of heightened attentiveness to reality (the here and now). Putting themselves in harmony with the *dao*, their activities become imbued with purpose, since they eschew all action born of selfish desire as ineffectual and unillumined. The astute reader will recognize a similarity between *wu-wei* (not-doing) in the Daoist tradition and the desireless action outlined in the *Bhagavad Gītā*. The Dao, like Brahman, gives birth to all beings, sustains them, and then welcomes them back to the formless. The Daoist aspires to create without possessing, for when the fruits of actions are renounced, the master is freed from all taints of selfhood, and he spontaneously honors the Dao (which is hidden but always present).

The *Secret of the Golden Flower*, a mystical Daoist text that circulated orally before being recorded in the eighteenth century, contains an interesting fusion of religious and philosophical Daoism with alchemy. The unknown author of this recondite manuscript recognizes that there are "very many alchemical teachings, but all of them make temporary use of effort to arrive at effortlessness." Due to that inherent shortcoming, "they are not teachings of total transcendence and direct perception." Contrarily, the "golden flower" technique of turning the light of consciousness around represents a return to the "absolutely real energy" of the Dao. This inner alchemy transmutes ordinary consciousness into that of a Daoist mystic, which metaphorically speaking is the "same thing as the gold pill" of immortality.[34]

Lesser alchemists mistake the symbols (the substances in the physical world combined to make pure gold out of dross) for the spiritual reality to which Daoist texts such as *The Secret of the Golden Flower* attest; the extrapolation of gold from base metals is only important to those bent on riches in this world. Distilling the celestial mind out of ordinary egoic consciousness, by contrast, is accomplished by turning the light of the mind inward, so as to become aware (in each moment) of the coming and going not just of mental forms, but those in the material world as well. In the still point of the center, one becomes "detached" or "free" from all phenomena, yet remains pristinely aware of their appearance and disappearance.

Understandably, it might disappoint some readers that the "golden flower" is not a celestial cannabis tree that magically bestows healing and purified vision on the earnest partaker. The alchemical art of "turning the light around" requires attentive vigilance *at all times* until the elixir distills in the chamber of the mind; then a shift (or transmutation) takes place in consciousness after which attention rests in awareness effortlessly. That process is described in the *Secret of the Golden Flower*:

> Ordinarily, once people let their eyes and ears pursue things, they get stirred up, only to stop when things are gone. This activity and rest are all subjects, but the sovereign ruler becomes their slave. This is "always living with ghosts."
>
> Now if in all activity and rest you abide in heaven in the midst of humanity, the sovereign is then the real human being. When it moves, you move with it; the movement is the root of heaven. When it is at rest, you rest with it; the rest is the moon cavern.[35]

After long, hard work, the pure attention of consciousness rises up into "the chamber of *the creative*." With the light of the spirit focused unremittingly on one's thoughts and actions in the world of time, one masters the ability to stay "awake" and not be taken away by thought or occurrence. Then, in "utter quiescence, not a single thought is born."[36] That moment of transfiguration of consciousness is the real thaumaturgy, the inner alchemy, of religious Daoism. Pure gold stands for the light of the focused mind; the golden flower represents the process of unfolding that is awakening.

From these social, medical, and alchemical references to cannabis in the Chinese tradition, we turn to Tibet—the rooftop of the world—for a final illustration of marijuana medicine in Asia utilized to heal the body and as an aid in spiritual practice. On the Tibetan plateau, straddled by India to the west and China to the east, massive open skies meet the jagged peaks of the Himalayas. Averaging more than 4,250 meters (nearly 14,000 feet) above sea level, the sunlight falling there possesses a singular vivid immediacy that illumes everything seemingly from within. In that expansive, arid, and rugged land, a person may sometimes see hundreds of kilometers into the distance. Due to its importance, Tibet has always hosted visitors, merchants, mendicants, and doctors from India and China. Some of those who crisscrossed its mountains and valleys left behind knowledge of their religio-medical traditions for posterity, and over time those understandings mixed (sometimes seamlessly) with indigenous shamanistic and animistic Bön traditions.

Human life can be difficult to sustain in such an unforgiving climate and on that challenging terrain, and to assist in that effort the people of Tibet envisioned a host of animistic spirits who filled the natural world. Some of them (such as ancestors' spirits) were regarded as potentially beneficial to human beings while others were necessarily injurious—but they all required ritual propitiation. In the native Tibetan Bön tradition, boundaries between the living and the spirit worlds were highly porous, and funeral services included sacrifices, food offerings, and the entombment of corpses with precious objects thought of use to the soul in the afterlife. Bön retains a distinctive self-conscious religious identity today, albeit one shaped by many foreign religious and philosophical traditions (including Chinese, Hindu, and Buddhist).

This intersection of traditions in Tibet made possible the formulation of a unique form of Buddhism known as Vajrayāna (or Tantra). The word

"Tantra" connotes a "weaving together" of Indian Vedānta, Shaivite Hinduism, and a pantheon of Bön deities with an arcane knowledge of medical herbs. While Chinese contributions to Vajrayāna medicine were significant, they remained secondary to those of Ayurveda. However, botanicals played an important role in both Chinese and Ayurvedic medicine, and the abundance of cannabis growing wild in the Tibeto-Himalayan region meant that healing herb was readily accessible. Its seeds were used to make cooking oil, but the remaining parts of the plant were dedicated to the treatment of skin and lymph disorders, the repair of slow healing wounds, and the maintenance of overall vitality. Other common applications of cannabis in Vajrayāna medicine include the treatment of paralysis of the tongue, convulsions, breaking up phlegm, and the termination of delirium during fever.[37]

Although, strictly speaking, the Tantric use of cannabis commences in the seventh century, Vajrayāna originated in India and is associated with Shaivism (and the Vedic soma cults that preceded it). Therefore, Tantric practitioners may lay claim to a legacy of cannabis use that begins with references to bhang (bhaṅgā) in the Rig Veda and Atharva Veda. This identification with sacred Indian traditions is so great that Tantric scripture is sometimes referred to as the "Fifth Veda" (the Atharva Veda being commonly regarded as the fourth).[38] In their emulation of Indian Tantra, some Vajrayāna Buddhists consume bhang to lower inhibitions during occult sexual practices believed to facilitate religious awakening. The socially transgressive nature of some of those observances, including the ritual ingestion of body fluids, reminds one of the Sādhus in India who unabashedly reject dominant social mores by eating taboo foods and violating cherished values. Buddhist Tantra (sometimes known as esoteric Buddhism) integrated established Indian practices such as mantra, mandala, soma, and fire sacrifices and developed them into a comprehensive religious system.[39]

Vajrayāna mantra practice involves a repetition of sounds to access alternate states of consciousness, while mandala practice emphasizes intense visualization of complex geometric patterns in the ritual object. A mandala is a geometric art form of "center and circle" drawn, painted, or made of colored sand, and used for meditation. The mandala symbolizes enlightened body, mind, and speech, and sometimes serves as a preventative and curative therapeutic through which a natural state of primordial purity may be glimpsed in order to speed healing. A Tibetan monk undertaking such an exercise might stare into a mandala while in seated meditation, or make it a model for visualizations whereby the mandala is imagined as a palace filled with deities. Such a "perfect place" requires focused imaginative exploration through mindful cognition, and the meditator is the sole hero therein (with his body envisioned as the mandala deity).[40] Some mandala exercises resemble the mnemonic "memory palace" technique used by the Italian Jesuit Matteo Ricci, but Tantric practices aim to quicken spiritual liberation (rather than simply strengthen memory).

Notwithstanding its unapologetic accommodation of religious practices such as mandala, mantra, and sacrifice, Tibetan Vajrayāna remains fundamentally a Buddhist tradition. The venerable saint Atīśa (b. 980), who helped to spread Buddhism in Tibet, acknowledged three different methods of practice in the pursuit of spiritual insight: samadhi (concentration or insight), *sūtrayāna* (scriptural study), and *Tantrayāna* (Vajrayāna or mysticism).[41] Vajrayāna thereafter became known as a vehicle for deliverance by way of realization of an indivisible divine principle that cannot be grasped by conceptualization or ratiocination. Tantric liberation relies upon the integral interrelationships between mind and body, an important feature of the Asian healing arts more generally, and its methods allow for herbal elixirs in the quest for realization.[42] In this respect, early Vajrayāna Buddhist *materia medica* shares more with Ayurveda, and other approaches developed alongside it, than with traditional Chinese medicine.

We close this chapter, not with bhang-imbibing monks at their esoteric tantric rites, but with Jamgön Mipham's *Dispelling Darkness of the Ten Directions*, a commentary on the famed *Tantra of the Secret Essence* (*Guhyagarbha-tantra*) dedicated to revealing the numinous mind of wisdom for mental and physical healing. To demonstrate that reality is perceived in accordance with one's mental state, the text illustrates the extent to which deluded thinking transmogrifies the world into a wasteland. Self-absorption and depression lend to nature a pale cast, but with an empty quiet mind, "pure appearances will faultlessly dawn."[43] Until one reaches that state of permanent "reversal" whereby confused appearances are abandoned—and pure appearances are put in tune with reality once and for all—perception will vacillate between these two poles.

To illustrate this point, readers of the *Tantra of the Secret Essence* are asked to consider an uncongealed mass formed out of coarse earthen gold, but mixed with fine gold and quicksilver (coal, water, and herbal ingredients). To "confused" individuals who remain unaware of the transformative potential of that mass to become pure gold when heated, that mass will simply appear to be a glob of fresh butter. Wise individuals who gaze upon the same butter-like mass will immediately "perceive its ability to appear in various ways depending upon the various conditions that it meets with." This notion of perception varying according to spiritual insight underscores the importance of establishing an abiding shift in consciousness—the intended outcome of alchemical transformation of the self:

> When such a mass is cold, it will remain like a mass of fresh butter for an extremely long time. When it touches a flame and heats up, however, it will become the color of copper, bronze, and brass. Likewise, when heated with a strong flame, it will become the nature of ordinary gold, and will become the nature of the finest gold when heated thoroughly. From that point on, it will not change in nature, no matter what temperature its surroundings are.[44]

In a similar way, when the mind is put in continual accord with reality, false appearances become purified and freed of egoic blemish. As for the consciousness of others, Jamgön Mipham Rinpoche concludes that we should just "accept that those of us with impure minds and impure eyes perceive things in an impure manner."[45] However, he sensibly asserts that if everyone experienced pure appearances (true perception) there would be nothing more about which to argue or write.

In this chapter, we followed a cannabis trail out of India, the Middle East, and Central Asia, through Tibet, and into China (where the practical applications of hemp eclipsed its psychoactive properties). Continuing onward to the African continent, we take stock of arresting correspondences pertaining to the ways in which ancient and medieval peoples utilized cannabis across the globe. Chapter 4 opens with the ancient Egyptians but moves quickly to the Early Modern period (c. 1500–1800) in order to follow dagga cults into southern Africa and kef northwestward along the coast toward Morocco. After illustrating the perennial nature of peak-experiences in Mediterranean mystery cults and Native American shamanism, chapter 6 brings this spiritual history to a close with scientific and literary explorations of cannabis in Europe and the Americas from the Renaissance to the twenty-first century.

4

DAGGA CULTS, COPTIC CHURCHES, AND THE RASTAFARI

Whether speaking of the diversity of its flora and fauna or the multiplicity of its peoples, languages, histories, and cultures, no other region of the globe presents researchers with the complexity of Africa. Early hominids separated from primates from 4 to 10 million years ago on the continent, followed by Australopithecus 3.5 million years ago, the tool-wielding *Homo habilis* a million years later, and then the taller bipedal *Homo erectus*.[1] While theories of multiple origin (multiregionalism) continue to garner critical attention, scholarly consensus suggests that *Homo sapiens* emerged in Africa some 250,000 years ago, sporting the larger brains that enabled them to better exploit the natural environment to build shelters, gather food resources, and fabricate tools for hunting and fishing (an achievement perfected only twelve thousand years ago).[2]

Seven to eight millennia ago, the Sahara Desert was covered with tall trees and lush green meadows, and in that haven settlers first began to build semipermanent agricultural habitations, thus interrupting the migration patterns of hunter-gatherers whose lifestyles were built around meager subsistence. Perceiving the advantages offered by more permanent dwellings and the regular cultivation of the land, African peoples progressively learned to settle and tend livestock. Their harvests of cereal grains and regular access to milk from domesticated animals significantly increased the amount of protein in their diets, making more complex forms of settlement and social organization possible. As the climate changed around 3000 BCE, the Sahara became arid and uninhabitable, and so human beings migrated southward, northward, and eastward toward the Nile River—the site of the continent's first major civilization, known as "Kemet" to Africans and "Egypt" to the Greeks.

The longest river in the world, the Nile once ran unobstructed and graced the inhabitants of its basin with seasonal flooding so perfectly coinciding with planting cycles that some farmers had only to sow seeds in the soft earth (after waters receded) and allow livestock to trample them into the soil. Such abundant fertility made possible the experiment at Kemet, the first instance in human history of individuals organizing themselves into a nation composed of different ethnic and social communities.[3] A country of peasants, farmers, civil servants, tax collectors, and scribes, the ancient Kemetic peoples honored as gods animal spirits and the forces of nature (usually in triads). In their religious practices, they venerated divinities such as Ra (the sun god), Nun (the god of the primordial waters), Shu (god of the air), and the Ibis (a symbol for Tehuti—conferrer of the gifts of writing, mathematics, language, and magic to human beings). The citizens of Kemet obeyed a deified king recognized as an incarnation of one of many gods, and an obsequious priesthood buttressed that supposition of divinity and provided the sovereign with political backing.[4]

According to the ancient funerary text best known as the *Egyptian Book of the Dead*, which contains spells and charms to assist the deceased in navigating the underworld, there was only nonbeing at the beginning of time. Out of that nothingness came Ptah, the master architect of the universe, and his emanations produced the trinity of Osiris, Isis, and Horus.[5] Egyptian myths, such as this one, provided the foundation for a shared African philosophy of origins and helped to establish credulity in the divine nature of kingship, which justified indigenous African models of theocratic government and sacred monarchy traceable in other African kingdoms (such as those in Nigeria, Zimbabwe, and South Africa). Traditionally, it rationalized social and political hierarchies and a centralized model of governance in which power always flowed downward.[6]

Historians distinguish nearly thirty ancient Egyptian dynasties from approximately 3000 to 300 BCE. Over that extensive period, wisdom literatures, medical and mathematical treatises, and poetry and priestly rituals were recorded following the innovation of writing in Egypt (perhaps as early as 3400 BCE, a scant three hundred years before the development of cuneiform in Mesopotamia).[7] They wrote in order to memorialize historical events, preserve literary and didactic works, and facilitate communication between kings, priests, and scribes. The master masons of Egypt built monumental pyramids and carved giant sphinx protector figures for the royal dead,[8] and their artists painted in an unmistakable style that still captures the imaginations of museumgoers around the globe (who rush to see gold funerary items, mummies, and sculptures from this important African civilization).

Although only fragments remain from the earliest Egyptian medical papyruses, and most of the names of the plants featured in their medical formulas elude botanical identification, *Cannabis sativa* was among the florae cataloged in that pharmacopoeia. The recent identification of the ancient Egyptian word for "hemp" (Šmšmt) made possible the decipherment of pyramid inscriptions that revealed a variety of medical uses for the plant, including as a topical oil and ointment for inflammation.[9] Ancient Egyptians made rope from hemp, and a reasonable possibility exists for their ritual and recreational consumption of cannabis, as high concentrations of THC have been measured in at least nine Egyptian mummies. Although doubt has been cast upon these results, in addition to mandrake and opium poppy, ancient Egyptians "used Indian hemp as a sedative and as a spasmolytic agent."[10]

Once it had fallen into dynastic decline, Egypt endured continual foreign invasion and occupation. Alexander the Great invaded in 332 BCE, and Roman rule of that land reached an apex six hundred years later. Christianity took root in Egypt within a hundred years of the crucifixion of that tradition's founder, and it would endure despite the Muslim conquests that spread Islam across the African continent from the seventh century onward. These complex overlays of indigenous beliefs, European Christianity, and Arab Islam lend the African people an array of cultural ideas upon which to draw.[11]

The oldest Christian churches in Africa are located in Egypt and Ethiopia and date from the first century. The supreme head of the Coptic churches, called pope, is the patriarch at Alexandria and said to be a direct successor to St. Mark the Evangelist. As the early Christian church took shape, clerics and scholars in Egypt became instrumental in debating major tenets and framing fundamental beliefs. By the fourth and fifth centuries, that movement formulated its own trinity (in the Father, Son, and Holy Ghost) and affirmed faith in a glorious afterlife. The indigenous pharaonic triune of Osiris, Isis, and Horus provided a recognizable symbolic framework for the conversion of the masses to the new religion. [12]

In that context of religious transition, a sect of early Gnostic Christians is notable for the buried treasure trove of more than fifty religious manuscripts (arranged in thirteen codices) that it left to posterity. An Arab laborer inadvertently discovered that collection in 1945 while digging for fertilizer around a fieldstone near Nag Hammadi in upper Egypt. The manuscripts reveal much about the doctrinal struggle for orthodoxy that played out during the first few hundred years of Christian history. Deemed heretical by a burgeoning ecclesiastical leadership for their emphasis on personal religious revelation, the Gnostics and their brand of mystical Christianity largely vanished by the late fourth century—about the time that the Nag Hammadi texts were carefully inhumed.

Adherents of Gnosticism read scriptures symbolically with an eye toward discovering hidden meanings (much as their Sufi counterparts did later with the Quran and other sacred writings). They envisioned God as a supreme oneness, rather than as a trinity or duality, and they tended to interpret the martyrdom of Jesus Christ in metaphorical terms of spiritual rebirth. Their rites offered initiates "gnosis," knowledge of spiritual mysteries and salvation through direct revelation. For these and other reasons, early Church fathers (who represented the institutional Christianity established to maintain order, articulate lines of authority, and safeguard stability) saw the Gnostic brand of individual salvation as a serious threat to the role that they desired for themselves as intermediaries between believers and their God. Consequently, they attacked with all their fervor, throwing charges of heresy at Gnostic schools, which organically developed at the intersection of Christianity, Neoplatonism, and indigenous religions. [13]

The Nag Hammadi texts demonstrate that the Gnostics developed a vision of humanity and human society that bordered on the utopian. From their scriptures, painstakingly translated over decades, we understand their Jesus as a guide to personal salvation, rather than a savior of all humankind. He revealed the way to self-knowledge through what were regarded as secret teachings preserved in the Nag Hammadi codices. Many of the surviving manuscripts reveal a very different inflection of Christian soteriology, one eclipsed by the rise of institutionalism as a means of social, economic, and political control. The intensely mystical tenor of their writings explains why some early Church fathers condemned the Gnostics as a dire threat to emergent Christian orthodoxy.

The Coptic Gnostic scriptures found at Nag Hammadi include works such as *The Thunder: Perfect Mind*, *The Gospel of Truth*, *The Gospel of Thomas*, and *The Gospel of Mary* (Magdalene). *The Thunder: Perfect Mind* is a mystical discourse narrated by an unidentified female. Its paradoxical exhortations from the first person point of view are best conceived as part of a Judeo-Christian tradition of "wisdom" literatures that includes *Job*, *Psalms*, *Proverbs*, and *Ecclesiastes*. The arresting first lines of *The Thunder: Perfect Mind* are quoted at some length to give readers a sense of their force:

> I was sent forth from the power,
> and I have come to those who reflect upon me,
> and I have been found among those who seek after me.
> Look upon me, you who reflect upon me,
> and you hearers, hear me.
> You who are waiting for me, take me to yourselves.
> And do not banish me from your sight.
> And do not make your voice hate me, nor your hearing.
> Do not be ignorant of me anywhere or anytime. Be on your guard!
> Do not be ignorant of me.

> For I am the first and the last.
> I am the honored one and the scorned one.
> I am the whore and the holy one.
> I am the wife and the virgin.
> I am [the mother] and the daughter.
> I am the members of my mother.
> I am the barren one
> and many are her sons.
> I am she whose wedding is great,
> and I have not taken a husband.
> I am the midwife and she who does not bear.
> I am the solace of my labor pains.
> I am the bride and the bridegroom,
> and it is my husband who begot me.
> I am the mother of my father
> and the sister of my husband
> and he is my offspring.
> I am the slave of him who prepared me.

I am the ruler of my offspring.
But he is the one who [begot me] before the time on a birthday.
And he is my offspring in time,
and my power is from him.
I am the staff of his power in his youth
and he is the rod of my old age.
And whatever he wills happens to me.
I am the silence that is incomprehensible
and the idea whose remembrance is frequent.
I am the voice whose sound is manifold
and the word whose appearance is multiple.
I am the utterance of my name. [14]

In the mystical vision of the poem, all oppositions, all conceptual judgments, and all dualities are eradicated through the use of contradictory assertions that give expression to the ineffable.

In *The Gospel of Mary*, Jesus offers Magdalene a direct revelation of the divine, an act of mercy implying that he loves her more than his other disciples, particularly Peter and Andrew (who represent orthodoxy in this gospel). In this fragmentary text, written sometime in the second century, Peter declares to Mary: "Sister, we know that the Savior loved you more than the rest of women. Tell us the words of the Savior which you remember—which you know (but) we do not, nor have we heard them." Mary responds that she "saw the Lord in a vision," and he told her: "Blessed are you, that did not waver at the sight of me. For where the mind is, there is the treasure." This revelation releases her from "the fetter of oblivion which is transient," and thereafter she attains to "the rest of the time, of the season, of the aeon, in silence." [15] These excerpts from *The Gospel of Mary* and *The Thunder: Perfect Mind* provide strong evidence of a Coptic Gnostic threat to a fledgling patriarchal orthodoxy during the first four hundred years of Christian church history.

In the wake of doctrinal orthodoxy from the fourth and fifth centuries onward, most devotees abandoned Gnostic beliefs and turned instead to institutions such as the Ethiopian (or Abyssinian) Church. However, the successful excision of Gnosticism from Christendom (for its emphasis on personal revelation and openness to a variety of unmediated religious experiences) came at a cost: a series of schisms that split off Eastern Orthodox Christianity from the rest of the Church. One early rift took place after Emperor Constantine embraced Christianity as a bulwark of the imperial system during the fourth century. The first ecumenical Council of Nicaea, called by Constantine, adopted the creed that Jesus was God and consubstantial with the Father. The subsequent Council of Chalcedon affirmed the human and divine nature of Jesus, which led to the formation of Coptic Christianity (sans Gnosticism) as an expression of Egypt's separatist religious identity—and in opposition to Rome and Constantinople as seats of Church authority over Alexandria. [16]

Despite the rise of mainstream Coptic Christianity, a long tradition of desert monasticism endured in Africa that sanctioned religious contemplation in isolation from the world. During this period, many Christian ascetics in Egypt and Ethiopia smoked cannabis from ornamental pipes in order to bolster their fortitude during ritual fasts, mortifications, and vigils. [17] The use of the Coptic language, into which the Nag Hammadi texts were translated from Greek, continued until the arrival of Islam, but it went into steady decline in the eleventh century as Egyptian and Ethiopian writers began using Arabic (although Coptic does survive today). The Arab invasion of Ethiopia ended in the destruction of more than three thousand Christian churches, and many Copts were forced to relinquish their faith during the rule of the Fatimid caliphs from the tenth to twelfth centuries. Coptic Christians suffered terribly under some medieval Mamluk rulers, as well.

Cannabis, on the other hand, spread quickly across the continent along with the expansion of Islam, for the plant remained an important psychoactive agent in the medieval Muslim world, and it continued to be credited with opening deeper levels of perception. [18] Mystic devotees from Syria planted cannabis in Egypt during the mid-twelfth century, and they employed it in religious and communal settings to increase sociability, activate intelligence, stir jocularity, and encourage meditativeness. [19] Its prevalence led the thirteenth-century Spanish historian Ibn Sa'īd al-Maghribī to bewail hashish consumption in Egypt, and his contemporary, the physician Ibn al-Bayṭār, reported seeing Sufis in that country eating baked cannabis leaves (with honey or rolled into paste pills). [20]

Over the next several hundred years, European colonists, mercenaries, merchants, and missionaries invaded the continent, but through it all, the Egyptian people managed to preserve sufficient cultural continuity to forge a shared national identity during the postcolonial era—and Egypt remains a land of cannabis enthusiasts to this day. Cannabis continued its journey to other regions of Africa, despite various attempts to brand the herb a menace. As it traversed that continent, it was increasingly blended with native herbs and formed into powders and pastes for eating, inhaling, or smoking. In fact, long prior to the introduction of cannabis, plant medicines featured prominently in a wide variety of ritual and medical contexts across Africa, and traditional pharmacopoeias included consciousness-altering substances for the diagnosis and treatment of disease.[21]

Hard and fast distinctions between religious ritual and medical practice did not exist in many indigenous cultures, and African shamans are another example of native medical practitioners given to mysticism who were authorized by their peers to practice herbal medicine, divination, invocation, magic, and prayer. They administered psychoactive decoctions in the form of enemas, snuff, or oral doses and listened attentively to the uninhibited narratives of medicated patients for clues concerning the origins of their illnesses.[22] Among the Igbo people of Nigeria, for instance, shamans worked as healers of the body and mind, and they enforced sacred laws, participated in tribal governance, and acted as educators in the community.[23] In addition, they availed themselves of herbs and certain barks that induced peak-experiences,[24] a practice that speaks to a natural human propensity for transpersonal meaning-making through alternate states of consciousness.

In addition to its role in inducing shamanistic ecstasy, cannabis found an important place in community rituals designed to evoke spirits of the ancestors and placate them with its sweet incense. The inclusion of shamans in ceremonial rites helped to ensure social stability and the prosperity of community members. In southern Africa, where the plant is known as dagga (a term of Arabic or Khoikhoi origin whose variations include *dacha*, *dakkha*, *dacka*, or *daggha*), cannabis smoking is particularly prominent. In western Africa, cannabis is called *diamba* (*deiamba* or *riamba*), while in the east-central region of the continent, it is *bangi* (from the Sanskrit *bhaṅgā*).[25] Such variations in nomenclature provide another perspective on the spread of cannabis from India to Africa alongside Arab merchants and religious mendicants. In our own time, hemp is cultivated all over Africa as a fiber, textile, and medicine—as well as a pleasant intoxicant.

The term "dagga" (and its variants) sometimes refers to an assortment of psychoactive plants, including datura and "wild dagga" (*Leonotis leonurus*).[26] Generally speaking, however, cannabis quickly replaced many native medical agents, since it was not disadvantaged by undesirable side effects associated with more potent plant substances. Bantu-speaking tribes particularly valued it as a cure-all—finding cannabis effectual in treating asthma, malaria, blood poisoning, snakebites, and a host of other maladies. Believed to encourage aggressiveness on the battlefield and efficiency at work, Zulu peoples in South Africa smoked cannabis from gourd water pipes before entering a conflict or undertaking arduous tasks.[27]

The Khoikhoi people (sometimes disparagingly known as Hottentots) migrated to southwestern Africa sometime in the sixth century with herds of cattle and flocks of sheep. The Khoikhoi adhered to a patriarchal social order, and their language was distinguished by the use of click sounds. Villages were the traditional jurisdiction of chieftains whose powerful hereditary positions ensured harmony among tribal members and provided the political stability to work communally. The Khoikhoi trained oxen for skirmishes over land rights, which inevitably arose among semi-nomadic peoples who relied on the ability to move freely. When war came, guerilla tactics were generally considered more effective than launching pitched battles where the loss of life might be much greater.

In the hunt for wildlife, Khoikhoi men used a combination of spears, bows, and poisoned arrows to bring down prey (rather than deplete their own herds for sustenance), while women gathered food resources such as berries and nuts. Khoikhoi tribes traditionally lived in beehive shaped grass huts, built with flexible poles to form ceiling arches that were easily set up or struck down. Fiber blinds provided convenient access to the huts, the floors of which were covered with rugs or mats; household deities and daily use items lent an air of domesticity to sometimes-make-shift structures. Residential huts were generally arranged in a circle to create a community space at the center of the village, though that area also protected livestock from attack and harsh environmental conditions. Due to the hot climate, the Khoikhoi required only modest apparel, which took the form of decorative aprons, cloaks and capes, sandals, and fly-whisks formed from natural fibers and furs. Bead necklaces and head-dresses added adornment on ceremonial occasions.

In the evenings, the Khoikhoi gathered around crackling fires to exchange stories and make merry. To facilitate jocularity, a narcotic drink made from herbs and honey was served—and tobacco, dagga, and other aromatic herbs smoked—to enhance the preferred pastimes of song, dance, and music making with gourd instruments and reed pipes.[28]

Khoikhoi religious practices included honoring the moon with dances and a belief in three supernatural beings: a beneficent creator and controller of all good things, an oppositional being who oversaw all unpleasant events and distasteful manifestations in nature, and an ancestral hero-magician believed to have died many times and been buried in numerous places marked by piles of funerary stones.

In their cultural traditions, religion, ritual, magic, and medicine seamlessly melded. Shamans discerned the causes of illness and misfortune, cured the bewitched, and brought rain. Diviners collected plant and animal substances, which they made into medical formulas given orally, applied as poultices, or used topically.[29] Sadly, from the seventeenth century onward, Khoikhoi culture suffered disintegration and dislocation for a variety of reasons, including pressure from white colonialism, the encroachment of Bantu peoples, the ravages of smallpox, as well as absorption by the Xhosa Nation and other minority communities in southwest Africa.

Similarly surrounded by more established states (including the Xhosa, Sotho, and Swazi), the Zulu fought for prominence under the leadership of Shaka Zulu, a man believed to have murdered a half brother in order to gain the highest seat of authority. Shaka first served his tribe as a warrior, worked his way up to military commander, and eventually became chief of the clan (by usurping the rule of his brother). When he established leadership over that minor kingdom during the early nineteenth century, the Zulu people numbered in the hundreds, but under Shaka's tutelage they grew into a mighty military force. He expanded the Zulu nation by integrating ethnic groups as he conquered them and allowed vanquished leaders to submit and swear allegiance, or suffer summary execution. By recruiting young men and women and retaining them until they reached the age of thirty, Shaka swelled the ranks of the Zulu army. His introduction of rigorous discipline among the troops and invention of a highly effective short-stabbing spear (*assegai*), combined with innovations like the regiment as a unit of organization, led to a widespread belief in the near invincibility of Zulu warriors.[30]

When the whites came, the Zulu nation refused to live under their yoke, as so many African tribes had done after unsuccessfully challenging the deadly mechanized weaponry of the European forces. One cause for the increasing militancy of the Zulu was a colonial insistence that land and water resources could be bought and sold (an idea embedded in a cherished notion of private property in the West). Shaka's reign endured for just twelve years, but an estimated 1 million souls lost their lives or were left homeless as a result of his belligerence. Given that bloody reality, it may seem ironic that the word "Zulu" means "heaven." On the other hand, the Zulu understood that the earth could never belong to a single person or group—a sacred comprehension enshrined in an ancient African philosophy shared by the Xhosa, Tswana, Sotho, and Khoisan regarding land.[31]

The assassination of Shaka had already weakened the Zulu nation by the time Dutch Boer farmers moved into Zulu ancestral territory (in an effort to escape British domination farther south). The skillful warrior died in a manner similar to that which brought him to power; he was slain at the hands of his half brothers. Shaka's nephew Ceteswayo later again honed the Zulu army into a fighting force to be feared. The Zulu Declaration, adopted during the reign of Ceteswayo and written to restore the flagging fortunes of that nation, is cited (in part) below in the context of spirituality and healing. Inspired by the martial discipline and single-minded purpose of Shaka, it offers a glimpse into the intense religious sensibility that connected the Zulu people with the natural world:

I am
I am alive;
I am conscious and aware;
. . . .
I am the face of humanity;
The face of humanity is my face.
I contemplate myself and see everything in me.
. . . .
My neighbor's sorrow is my sorrow
His joy is my joy.
He and I are mutually fulfilled when we stand by each other in moments of need.
His survival is a precondition of my survival.
That which is freely asked or freely given is love;
Imposed love is a crime against humanity.
I am sovereign of my life;
My neighbor is sovereign of his life;
Society is a collective sovereignty;
It exists to ensure that my neighbor and I realize the promise of being human.
I have no right to anything I deny my neighbor.[32]

Should neighbors or adversaries violate the terms of this elegant declaration, war was justified. For this reason, when white settlers began building fences and walls to keep the Zulu out of their traditional ancestor burial grounds, a deadly confrontation loomed on the horizon.

Curiously, it was a domestic dispute between a senior member of Ceteswayo's government and his wife that became the pretext for British aggression. When the luckless woman escaped to the British section of Natal, a clumsy retrieval attempt resulted in her death. Usually the Zulu handled such sordid affairs internally, but eager for any excuse to attack, the British found one in Ceteswayo's refusal to surrender the guilty official. In January 1879, the British invaded Zululand; taken by surprise, the Zulu army suffered significant losses.[33] Near Isandlwana Mountain, however, Ceteswayo and his Zulu warriors struck back with great rapidity and deadly accuracy. Brandishing Shaka's short-stabbing spear, they sliced at the opposition until the battlefield rang with the cries of men missing arms, legs, and whose innards spilled out onto the ground. The Zulu policy of taking no prisoners made it easy for their colonial enemies to label them bloodthirsty monsters. Yet, after defeating nearly 2,500 British soldiers (along with their African troops), the Zulu killed those writhing in agony as an act of kindness, for they thought that even vicious foes should be spared the shame of an agonizing death.[34]

According to popular lore, Zulu warriors ingested cannabis before going into battle as a way to vanquish fear, but the war medicines that they smoked often contained admixtures of other herbs. Although the potency and efficacy of such battlefield medicines were likely overstated, Zulu men smoked herbs recreationally in the evening, and the Zulu people ingested cannabis in all its forms: the flowers and resin were inhaled for pleasure, the stalks and roots constituted some medicines, and beverages formulated from the stalk and root of the hemp plant were consumed as a respiratory expectorant. In addition, the Zulus rubbed hemp leaves into cuts, used the flowers to treat coughs, and made liquid decoctions with the plant to treat tuberculosis.[35] The savants of Zululand were dagga smokers who burned cannabis flowers through large water pipes. In times of crisis, these sages cured disease and prophesized the future—and perhaps as a consequence of that relationship to sagacity, cannabis continues to be associated with knowledge, discernment, and astuteness in southern Africa.

Renowned across the continent for their knowledge of plants, as well as for their compelling music, Pygmies constitute the largest and most diverse group of active hunter-gatherers, or forest foragers, in the world. The appellation "Pygmy," a Western term denoting race and sometimes regarded as deprecating, remains in wide usage. Anthropologists distinguish a score of unique Pygmy groups, among them the Tikar (in Cameroon), the Bambenga (in Congo), the Babinga (in Gabon), the Batwa (in Uganda), and the Twa (in Rwanda). Outstanding biological features among these groups include a shorter stature, wider noses, and thinner lips than people in nearby communities.[36] Often marginalized, discriminated against, and forced into subordinate positions, Pygmies see themselves as different from their neighbors, and they maintain mobile settlement patterns.

Although every Pygmy group is distinctive, cultural similarities permit several general observations concerning their lifestyles, cultural beliefs, and religious practices. For instance, members of Pygmy communities traditionally lived in gazebo-like huts made from woven ply stems and covered with leaves. The huts of individual families were once laid out in a circle, but that configuration eventually made way to a preference for semispherical structures built around more permanent rectangular shelters.[37] Able hunters, Pygmies employ a wide range of weapons suitable to their game; monkeys and large birds might be brought down with crossbows, while antelope and larger animals (including elephants) are hunted collectively with spears to the end of which are attached large blades. To supplement these hunting activities, Pygmies gather yams, nuts, mushrooms, leaves, and insects. Another one of their talents is locating honey—a skill that often requires a great deal of climbing. Some Pygmy groups living around large bodies of water, such as the BaTwa, fish occasionally, but otherwise that activity is not of prime importance to the community.[38]

Exceptionally fond of cannabis, Pygmies consume it before hunts to bolster their vigor and fortitude, though the discoveries of many psychoactive substances are attributed to them, such as the iboga root (*Tabernanthe iboga*) as a euphoriant.[39] Pygmies smoke cannabis from long reed pipes or water bongs fashioned from calabashes or clay, but pipes constructed from gourds, horns, earthenware containers, and even the ground are common throughout southern and central Africa.[40] Pygmy groups also offer another example of the beneficial relationship between cannabis and the musical arts. Famed for innovating a diversity of musical forms, Pygmy music combines polyphonic and contrapuntal singing with instrumental accompaniment (which rarely takes melodic leads). One might attribute the subtle intricacy of Pygmy music to the inspiration they draw from their rich forest soundscape. Their musical expressions include wordless yodeling, disjointed melodic phrases, and subpentatonic forms that combine to create highly textured compositions that invite the improvisation of musicians playing along on a variety of drums, gongs, musical bows, flutes, and harps. [41]

Pygmy music also reflects the egalitarian nature of its society (in which intermarriage is rare and cultural continuity valued), but the primary function of Pygmy music is prayer. The specialty professions of herb-gathering and music-making merge into religious worship during ceremonies in which spirits are contacted, divinations cast, and treatments for sorcery or misfortune made. Some group musical performances are designed to have a therapeutic healing effect on all members of the community. [42] While a typical Pygmy encampment consists of small numbers of coresident households, Pygmies consider the autonomy of the individual inviolable. For this reason, social hierarchies that plague most modern societies were never institutionalized. The Pygmy commitment to individual liberty also provides an overarching logic for all political relations, and community members are granted significant leeway in deciding where, and with whom, to live. As a result of the respect given to personal independence, competition between important members of the community never need take the form of coercive power. Elders, camp leaders, and other authority figures may freely dispense advice, but the decision to follow it rests with individual community members who possess a universal right of refusal. [43]

Similarly progressive attitudes exist among other African groups where cannabis is part of their daily lives. The Bena-Riamba, or "Sons of Cannabis," belong to a Bantu tribe of the Belgian Congo known as the Baluba. Although some accounts of this group remain dubious, it appears this dagga cult formed as a response to the political and social movements that took shape during the late nineteenth century (following regional disagreements regarding the presence of foreign traders in their territory). Eventually, the members of the Baluba who opposed that potentially dangerous foreign presence left to form another community on an adjacent riverbank. When King Kalamba Mukenge subsequently permitted the traders to enter, they brought with them the habit of smoking bhang that was already prevalent on the Zanzibar Coast.[44] Cannabis proved so popular among the members of his community that King Mukenge spurned the old fetishes of the tribes that he conquered, and united them all instead in regular ceremonial marijuana smoking.

If we can rely on the contemporaneous report of one Western observer, the elimination of old customs and the introduction of ritualized cannabis smoking transformed this Baluba sect significantly. They changed the name of their tribe to mark that renewal, prohibited the use of weapons in the village, ceased persecutions for witchcraft, and ended the sale of young girls by their parents. Religious ceremonies became so simplified that they were soon reduced to convening at night to smoke cannabis communally. In order to support such heavy consumption, the Bena-Riamba set aside extensive tracks of land for its collective cultivation,[45] while the king funded the essential administrative apparatuses of government by taking a fourth of all game hunted and levying a tax on caravan traders.

Once the Bena-Riamba adopted the custom of communal living, new ceremonial rituals took shape to welcome others into the tribe. Smoking impressive amounts of cannabis in public eventually became a social marker by which members distinguished themselves from nearby communities. According to one contemporary scholar, the Baluba smoke marijuana on all important festivals, and when concluding agreements and treaties of friendship, from large bottle gourds that could reach a meter in circumference.[46] While, admittedly, the thought of an intentional community of cannabis smokers is a startling proposition, these accounts of the Bena-Riamba are difficult to corroborate. Rather than become mired in that controversy, let us summarize several defining features of African religions relevant to our inquiry before moving on to the ascension of Emperor Haile Selassie in Ethiopia, who inadvertently inspired a motley band of cannabis-fueled rebels known as Rastafarians.

In Africa, the second largest continent after Asia and four times the size of the United States, seven hundred million souls practice a wide array of religious traditions in more than fifty countries. By limiting our observations to shared attitudes and practices among its indigenous cultures, several generalizations regarding fundamental belief structures may be ventured. Native African peoples believed that ancestor spirits acted in the world of the living, and that death simply marked a transition from one world to the next. Boundaries separating realms of the living, unborn, and dead—like those of the sky, human world, and the underworld—were envisioned as highly permeable, and their myths of creation focused around primordial beings who created humankind and imparted the essential skills of hunting and reproduction. Ritual practices built around sacred stories, gradually altered in the retelling over centuries (sometimes millennia), symbolically reenacted those narratives. [47]

Rather than holding fast to a linear sense of time (like that found in the Judeo-Christian-Islamic tradition with its Last Judgment), temporality is cyclic and coincides with patterns in the natural world. According to that worldview, every living and inanimate object is holy. Certain herbs tended to be venerated, and a comprehensive understanding of them remained a prerequisite for any diviner or priest. [48] In some African religious traditions, one finds a mystical belief in a numinous force that suffuses the cosmos. It usually displaces, but sometimes exists alongside of, ancestor and deity worship. According to such formulations, no inherent separation between mind and matter (or other ecological and cosmological influences in the human world) can exist, contrary to dualistic European religions. [49]

Instead, everything is endowed with an "animate-sentient-like" aspect, and therefore is alive on a fundamental level—rocks and stones pulsing with the same intense energy as every singing blade of grass and dancing bird. The earth is a living conscious organism—the universe, a single multidimensional and interpenetrating process. When reality is thus conceived as intersecting patterns of energies apprehended subjectively, all things are perceived as localized objects embedded in a web of relationships. [50] This recognition of the cosmos as a living entity, with the individual as an integral part, severs the illusory estrangement of egoic consciousness from the natural world—a source of great depression and anxiety in Western cultures. A similar dynamic matrix of vitality and energy informs African religious and healing practices as well, for that undifferentiated life force is thought to be amplified through prayer, invocations, praise songs, music, and dancing.

Due to the dynamic interpenetration of self and the physical world inherent in that nondual vision, the inner structure of things (and their relationship to corollary forces) may be manipulated by the consciousness of healer-sorcerers, who harness knowledge for good (while witchcraft implies their manipulation for nefarious ends). Well-intentioned indigenous healers in Africa gather herbs, plant them in their gardens, or purchase them in marketplaces. Some of them are potently mind-altering and therefore are given only with great care and considerable respect for their medical efficacy. The powers of herbs are augmented through healing rites, diet modifications, exercise or fasting, ceremonial sacrifices, and divinations. Traditional therapeutic rituals performed with proper intention are thought to increase the body's vitality by "tuning" it to that life force, and the natural herbs employed in traditional healing arts were part of that recalibration.

In transitioning to the Rastafarians in Jamaica, we understand that African tribes (including the Yoruba, Ankore, Igbo, Akan, and Shona) shared a vision of the universe as pulsating matrices of energies, which they brought to the New World when they were savagely enslaved.[51] Although chronicling those abuses remains beyond the scope of this project, we seek an understanding of the ways that African and Indian spiritual beliefs blended with Christianity in Jamaica—as well as an explanation for why the figure of Haile Selassie, the last reigning monarch of Ethiopia, so infectiously fired the zeal of Rastafarian movement founders.

For the ancient Greeks, the word "Ethiopian" designated all African peoples living to the south of Egypt. Unbeknownst to them, in that part of the world anatomically modern *Homo sapiens* first emerged before dispersing across the Middle East. Much later, sometime around 1000 BCE, the Kushite kingdom arose in the region known as Nubia (between modern day Egypt and Sudan). In order to avoid direct confrontation with Egypt, the dominant power in the region, the Kushite kingdom moved farther up the Nile where it flourished producing red ware, burnished black ware, and decorated cups with ankhs and stamped motifs. The Kush capital at Meroë became a leading trading center, reaching an apex between 1700 and 600 BCE. During that period, the Kush grew to rival Kemet (Egypt), its former colonizer. However, both kingdoms long benefited from mutual cultural and economic exchange.[52] The Kush fell to the Nobatae in the second century, but the Axumites would vanquish them just 150 years later.[53]

By the third century, the Ethiopian kingdom of Axum (or Aksum) was the most advanced civilization in Africa, and it superseded the Kushite kingdom as a center of philosophical thinking and writing. Soon thereafter, the Axumites became Christianized, and by the sixth century travelers commented on the number of churches and ecclesiastical positions already in place.[54] Christian monks in Ethiopia helped to preserve the unique organizational structures of Axumite Christianity—and their ascetics smoked cannabis from ornamental water pipes believing that it increased endurance for religious exercises, such as fasting.[55] The Axumite Empire endured for most of the first millennium, but it entered into decline with the arrival of Islam in the seventh century. Following the fall of the Axumite Kingdom, a Christian Zagwe dynasty survived until the thirteenth century. Countless Africans determinedly fought the brutal yoke of colonialism from the late-fifteenth century to the late-nineteenth century, but Europe's bloodthirsty colonial aspirations and military prowess remained unrivaled. The European trade in slaves, brutal massacres of local populations, and unquenchable lust for gold and other resources were too much for many indigenous peoples in Africa to withstand.

Although European colonists and Arab slave traders failed to completely subdue the African continent, they meted out some of the most brutal suffering ever inflicted on innocent people.[56] Joseph Conrad's novel *Heart of Darkness* chronicles the mass murder, enslavement, and unimaginable deprivation borne by the peoples of the Congo basin. Too often Christianity, as espoused by European missionaries, became an instrument of social and political control wielded by settler colonists—and thereby tacitly supported the slave trade and helped to justify its cruel violence. In the face of such sustained oppression, a new wave of African Christian churches (many of them Ethiopian) supported a determined spirit of resistance to foreign missions and colonial land-grabs. We keep in mind this intersection of history, culture, and religion in Ethiopia particularly, but in Africa more generally, to best understand the first Rastafarians—members of the Jamaican underclass who were predominantly descended from slaves and indentured servants.

Traditionally, Ethiopian kings derived their legitimacy through claims of direct descent from King Solomon of Israel and the Queen of Sheba (as well as the lineage of notable Axumite kings). These Solomonic rulers, ecclesiastically appointed by a Coptic bishop, were heads of government, as well as heads of the Church. In this manner, they secured a historical and religious justification to rule, and their power was respected. According to a national myth, an unbroken lineage of 230 rulers—from the first son of Solomon and Sheba (Menelik I) to Haile Selassie—exercised power in Ethiopia for nearly three thousand years. However, historical evidence points toward several interruptions of Solomonic rule, as well as of conscious attempts to reassert a narrative of historical continuity in the fourteenth century (following hundreds of years of dominance by the rival Zagwe dynasty).

Nevertheless, Ethiopian rulers fought off invading Arab, Turkish, and Italian armies over the centuries. Ras Makonnen, for example, the governor of Harar and father of Tafari Mäkonnen (Emperor Haile Selassie), played a leading role in defeating Italian forces at the Battle of Adowa in 1896. Following that remarkable victory over an imperial European foe by an African nation, Ethiopia grew into a beacon of self-determination for people around the world. The Pan-African movement that sprang out of that military triumph aimed to unite the African people in an effort to decolonize the continent, end racial discrimination and political injustice, and enforce human rights. In Jamaica, members of the oppressed underclasses also looked to Africa, and especially Ethiopia, with hope as they innovated a new creed of self-actualization based in part on African models of resistance to colonialism.

Long before Christopher Columbus spotted the island of Jamaica on his second voyage, and was marooned there on his fourth, the aboriginal Taino people inhabited Jamaica. Tragically, they all but disappeared within a few years of those first ominous encounters with the West as a result of disease, enslavement, and oppression by profit-seeking Europeans. The Spanish, in whose name Columbus claimed the island, settled Jamaica for approximately 150 years before the British gained control. Lawlessness characterized the early part of British rule, as pirates commanded the island's main port as a base from which to pillage other settlements in the Caribbean. During the eighteenth century, Jamaica attracted settlers eager to establish plantations to produce sugarcane (then known as "white gold"), but in order to make their large establishments profitable, colonists required an abundant supply of cheap labor—and so they imported slaves from colonial operations in Africa.

Those hapless individuals abducted from their homes and sold into slavery in Jamaica brought to the Caribbean some cultural features of their homelands, including their languages, religions, and musical traditions. They brought art, song, dance, and food traditions related to ceremonial rituals marking the human passage from birth to death too, along with respect for elders in the community and a heightened sensitivity to the natural processes of the earth and cosmos. An official census in 1800 affirms that the white population of Jamaica was just twenty thousand people, *while the black population on the island was estimated to be fifteen times as large.*[57] That disparity reveals the enormous reliance on slave importations required to make colonial plantation enterprises viable. When slavery was prohibited on the island in 1838, the sugar industry declined rapidly, though a boon in bananas and tourism followed. However, banana plantations also required considerable labor to operate, and so owners imported indentured laborers from India, Asia, and the Middle East following an outright ban on slavery.

Soon recognizing the need for more highly skilled workers in addition to physical laborers, British colonists began to educate the children of former slaves so that they might protect their private property, cultivate their land, and keep the plantation accounts.[58] In spite of this seeming improvement in work allotments, the families of freed slaves faced enormous challenges, including inadequate compensation (that kept ownership of private property out of reach), a high pole tax, limits on land ownership, and rampant racism. Uprisings, such as the Morant Bay Rebellion, underscored the harsh conditions faced by ex-slaves. Hundreds lost their lives when the white governor, Edward John Eyre, called in the militia to squash the rebellion and bring its leader, Baptist deacon Paul Bogle, to trial. Instead of just arresting the deacon as instructed, British troops murdered blacks indiscriminately and flogged hundreds more, set fire to thousands of homes, and then summarily sentenced and executed Bogle within a few hours of his arrest.

In this broad historical context of generational exploitation, we appreciate the distinctive features of the Rastafarian movement, and understand better how that group responded to oppression by a minority class. In a singular manner, the conspicuous ganja smoking and wild dreadlocked hairstyles of some Rastafarians signals a determined rejection of the British imperial culture that dominated Jamaica for centuries prior to the island's independence in 1962. The Rastafarian project necessitates the conscious reappropriation of a severed African heritage for the purpose of empowering the underclasses in Jamaican society—and to encourage the relinquishment of all cultural and psychological ties to the British (who disparaged African traditions and attempted to inculcate European mores among those islanders).[59]

Marcus Garvey, a native Jamaican, founded the Universal Negro Improvement Association (UNIA) in 1914, and he took his message of black pride, self-reliance, and political freedom to New York City where the

Harlem Renaissance was in full flowering contemporaneously with the noirist (black consciousness) movement in Haiti, Afro-Cubanism in Cuba, and Negritude in the French Antilles. Garvey endorsed the Pan-Africanism that would later gain recognition following the lights of George Padmore, Léopold Senghor, Aimé Césaire, and Jomo Kenyatta. Garvey gave credence to Christian beliefs, only from a black perspective, and the liberation ideology known as "Garveyism" featured an interweaving of religiosity (including indigenous and Judeo-Christian-Islamic features) with African nationalism. In these and other early twentieth-century movements for social justice, we observe a collective political struggle for deliverance from the manacles of racial inequality.

In an effort to inspire underprivileged members of the African diaspora in the Americas, and around the world, Garvey venerated mighty African kingdoms and proudly celebrated their many contributions to human history. He made clear that disparities in wealth among members of any society led to avarice, tyranny, murder, and sometimes genocide. Garvey ridiculed the prevailing "white-centric" point of view, which he sought to replace with an "afro-centric" one—that is, to put an African savior in place of a Caucasian Jesus. Convicted on charges of financial wrongdoing after more than ten years of community organizing in the United States, Garvey was deported to Jamaica in 1927, where he continued to spread his message.[60] Garvey preached that a king would soon be crowned in Africa who would redeem the lost tribes of Judah and call them home. Self-appointed preachers appeared on the streets of Kingston and other Jamaican cities about the same time, and they walked into a moment of renewed spiritual excitement within Jamaican Christian churches, which reached a peak in the African-Christian tradition known as Revival Zion (or Revivalism).

In contrast to local Revivalist leaders, who held outdoor meetings in urban centers of activity and in rural areas, wandering visionaries proclaimed their divine message on the mean streets of Jamaica. These itinerate street ministers came to a peculiar conclusion concerning the Ethiopian prince Ras Tafari (later crowned Emperor Haile Selassie I), but it was one attributable to a confluence of religious, cultural, and intellectual traditions that at once rejected colonial power and appropriated biblical messianism, the belief that a liberator would come to end the oppression of people everywhere.[61]

The coronation of Haile Selassie in 1930 seemed to confirm the prophecies of Garvey and the street preachers, who spotted numerous signs of the emperor's divinity, such as those in his formal ruling titles: "King of Kings," "Lord of Lords," and perhaps most impressively, "Conquering Lion of the Tribe of Judah." They remembered that Selassie contributed to the liberation of Ethiopia from Mussolini and the Italians through an intensive international press campaign, and to messianic-minded Jamaicans, that victory signaled that Prince Ras Tafari fulfilled the biblical prophecies regarding the lion of Judah and the beast in Revelation (verses 5:2–6 and 19:19).[62] Before long, Garvey and the street preachers were to proclaim the Ethiopian emperor Jesus Christ incarnate. Shortly thereafter Garvey attained prophetic status among the Rastafarians, but Haile Selassie was their messiah. Such a narrative provided them with the historical linkages needed to forge a new Jamaican identity—one that reveled in Africa's glorious past.

Some credulous Jamaicans subscribed to the erroneous belief that historians had verified Haile Selassie's throne as the oldest in the world (as well as a direct descendent of King Solomon and Queen of Sheba). Therefore, they assumed that the new emperor would help them to throw off the yoke of white and black oppression in Jamaica and elsewhere, a notion in keeping with their condemnation of the island's exploitative social hierarchies and colonial government. Before long, the Garvey message and the Afro-centric teachings of the street ministers were transmuted into an adoration of the Lord God, Jah Rastafari. This transition made possible the rapid spread of the Rastafarian movement throughout the Caribbean, but it also took hold in Britain, the United States, and urban West Africa.

The Rastafarian nation is therefore a diverse one, with many leaders, rituals, and religious convictions. Nevertheless, a set of central beliefs binds Rastafarians together: they see Babylon as a symbol of decadence and false religions, they find rampant idolatry of other gods appalling, and they condemn corrupting ideas as the enemy of the proper worship of Jah (an abbreviation for "Jehovah"). Rastafarians possess a keen reverence for nature and natural living, and this attitude toward the environment manifests itself in the production of organic foods grown in self-sufficient cooperatives that hark back to village lifestyles in Africa. In addition, Rastafarians imagine the whole world as potentially part of a single multiracial homeland called Ethiopia,[63] and they firmly believe that cannabis was given to mankind for the "healing of the nations" (Revelation 22:2). They cite Genesis 1:12 in support of their veneration of the holy herb: "And the earth brought forth grass, and herb yielding seed after his kind, and the tree yielding fruit, whose seed was in itself, after his kind: and God saw that it was good."

The biblical story of the liberation of the Israelites from slavery under the pharaohs by the prophet Moses also provided a locus around which to shape a distinctly Rastafarian identity. They imbued that narrative of freedom from Israelite oppression in Babylon with a conviction in the redemptive possibility of Ethiopia (much in the same way that the American Black Church appropriated tropes of redemption from the Bible). Rastafarians hold fast to the belief that the oppressive institutions of Babylon (Western bourgeois culture) will eventually fall, and Ethiopia will be reconstituted as a land of peace, love, and togetherness.[64] In Rastafarian theology, this utopian impulse is known as "Ethiopianism," an intellectual and cultural movement that harkens back to an idealized past.

Those aspirations for social amelioration were on display in Pinnacle, an intentional community established by Leonard Howell, one of the founders of the Rastafarian movement. At Pinnacle, families lived together in small huts, cultivated the plots of land apportioned to them, and contributed to community projects. They raised animals and grew crops such as beans, corn, various tubers, and of course plenty of marijuana. In fact, for decades Jamaica ganja was the preferred cash crop of the island—albeit an illegal one. The production and sale of that revered herb meant that Pinnacle attained near self-sufficiency (having even made a provision for early childhood education for all community members). Pinnacle proved a short-lived experiment that ended with police raids of the compound, and its eventual abandonment and demolition.[65]

The Rastafarian movement carried on, nonetheless, by jettisoning some of the features of Revivalism that initially enthused the group, but those changes were part of a natural process of differentiation by which the Rastafarians defined themselves against the status quo. Whereas early Rastas came largely from the African-Jamaican rural and urban underclasses, and their religious and cultural practices revealed features of the peasantry, the second generation of youthful Rastafarians turned more militant, and they quickly earned the ire of a government blindly following the unenlightened drug policies of the United States. This new generation of Rastafarians elevated ganja smoking to a sacred ritual, and they spurned razor blade and hair clippers in favor of tangled dreads and unkempt beards.

Although Garvey retained his prophetic status as the Rastafarian movement developed, his rejection of sacramental cannabis, combined with the fact that he ran a highly centralized organization in the UNIA and embraced nationhood (rather than repatriation to Africa). This rejection created a schism between Rastafarians advocating for a fundamental break with Western bourgeois culture and a black middle-class embrace of nationalist movements, such as Garvey's.[66] For these reasons, contemporary Rastafarian ideology was influenced by Garveyism but did not arise directly from it. Undeterred by the appearance of different sects (including Bobo Shanti, Twelve Tribes, and Nyahbinghi), Rastafarians continue to scorn authority, social hierarchies, and leaders making unilateral decisions on behalf of a community or nation. Their firm commitment to individual liberty and autonomy recalls the Pygmy creed referenced earlier.

In contrast to Garveyism, which basically died out as a movement in the twenty-first century, the Rastafarian nation, which epitomizes a determined denunciation of social injustice in the mode of the Hebrew prophets, has gone global. Reggae music, the best ambassador for the movement, is enjoyed by millions of people around the world, though few of them fully appreciate the religious, philosophical, and cultural beliefs that underpin it. In addition to the importance of Haile Selassie, the idealization of Ethiopia as the "Promised Land" (Zion), and an aspiration for repatriation (which peaked after the creation of Israel in 1948), the practice of "Rastaology" contains several key elements that deserve discussion, most notably: "InI consciousness," the philosophy of "livity," and "dread-talk."

"InI consciousness" means the realization of one's own divinity, and it affirms black dignity and agency and provides ideological cohesion in the absence of codified social hierarchies in Rastafari culture. This recognition of inner divinity makes one a Rastafarian, and the simple grace of that message generates an openness to members of all nations and ethnicities in the movement. InI consciousness imbues the Rastafarian with an ultra-individualism adamantly opposed to bureaucratic structures, an ideal so entrenched that many Rastas refuse to identify with any group—including those of fellow Rastafarians! As an expression of free will, some reject the honored place given to *kaya* claiming that after reaching a certain level of spiritual attainment smoking ganja is no longer necessary.

Deconstructing the "InI" formulation further, the "I" might be interpreted as referring simultaneously to Ras Tafari (Emperor Haile Selassie I), Jah the divine "I," and the divinity residing in the individual self. The "I in I" part of the construction evokes the Hindu emphasis on nonduality (of Ātman and Brahman) discussed in chapter 1. Moreover, the conscious "I" is aware of mystical union with Jah, and the seeing "eye" apprehends the fundamentally divine nature of all people and the natural world.[67] This highly reflexive feature of InI consciousness recalls the mystic Meister Eckhart's celebrated declaration: "The eye through which I see God is the same eye through which God sees me; my eye and God's eye are one eye, one seeing, one knowing, one love."[68] Not coincidentally, Reggae artist Bob Marley's 1977 album *Exodus* features a track titled "One Love," for InI consciousness is perennial.

The Rastafarian term "livity" implies a way of living originating from an understanding that human health and longevity result from eating the organic foods with which Jah filled the earth. As a result, many Rastafarians commit to vegetarianism and support "back to the land" impulses that laud an agrarian way of life. In this sense, Rastafarians anticipated "organic" and "locally grown" movements in the United States and elsewhere by shunning processed foods and all chemical additives. Babylon has a predilection for the artificial, superficial, and the unnatural, but livity inspires faith in the power of herbs to provide energy and speed healing, whether gathered from the wild or cultivated at home. For nearly all Rastafarians, cannabis is the supreme herb, and they ingest it as a medicine in tea and food, and give it a prominent place in ritual communal activities.

According to Jamaican folk belief, cannabis possesses many medical attributes: most notably fortifying the blood, warding off disease, and promoting good health and well-being as prophylactic and therapeutic. Many cannabis preparations are credited with allowing one to work longer, harder, and faster and with increased overall stamina and vigor. In tea or tonic form, the plant is credited with preventing constipation, treating gonorrhea, curing arthritis, improving vision, and even making children smarter. Resinous flowers find their way into soups and stews, while stalks and leaves are added to teas. Some boil cannabis leaves to make soup-broths, but they are also cooked like spinach and fed to children.

Traditionally, cannabis smoking marked one as a member of the lower classes in Jamaica, or it was considered an adolescent rite of passage, which one forsook with age or class ascendance. Today, among independently minded Rastafarians, marijuana smoking endures as an important social rite that encourages communal bonding. Its ritual inhalation helps to codify camaraderie and signals equality, belonging, friendship, and trustworthiness. [69]

Rastafarians smoke ganja in the form of cigarettes known as "spliffs," but they also "toke" from *chilams* and water pipes (sacred vessels called "chalices" suggestive of the Holy Grail). [70] While there is no limit to the amount of cannabis they may imbibe, Rastas scorn other intoxicants, including alcohol and manufactured drugs. For most Rastafarians, cannabis is tantamount to the Tree of Life given to human beings by a benevolent creator to ensure good health and mental clarity. According to one of the tradition's mythologies, the hemp plant first grew on the gravesite of Solomon, the wisest person of all, and therefore it remains irrevocably tied to contemplation and understanding. [71]

In the estimation of one scholar, the Ethiopian Zion Coptic Church in Jamaica may lay claim to a lineage reaching back to the earliest sects of Christianity (when that fledgling religion was practiced in Jerusalem before moving to Africa). However, members of the Ethiopian Zion Coptic Church differ from Rastafarians in their rejection of Haile Selassie's divinity, and adherents believe that marijuana was taken as part of the Last Supper. [72] Smoked communally, the herb sustains a celebration of fellowship and revelation, without the need for priests to serve as intermediaries between the devotee and God. For Rastafarians too, marijuana leads one out of the false consciousness of Babylon (consumerism, materialism, inequality, injustice, racism, and exploitation) and toward a discovery of the True Self, the divine "I" capable of self-direction. [73] Many of these attributes are the same ones by which society may be positively transformed.

Given the hallowed place of cannabis in Rastafarian culture, the fact that the Jamaican government just started moving toward decriminalization in 2015 is quite remarkable. Yet, the adamant antidrug stance of the U.S. government, which hardened in the 1980s, led to crackdowns on cannabis even in the remotest areas of that Caribbean island. The Rastafarians interpreted those ignoble incursions as another form of oppression (by keeping the sacred healing herb from religious members of the nation). For decades, prohibitions on the cultivation, sale, and distribution of cannabis prompted continuous strife between Rastafarians and Jamaican authorities, particularly during the Rastafarian militant period from the 1950s to 1970s. Now, perhaps at last, Rastafarians are "coming in from the cold."

As noted above, dreadlocks symbolize a rejection of Western market values and hierarchies privileging money, power, and classism. Global capitalism is regarded as a form of repression that exploits laborers to enrich multinational corporations. In their choice of hairstyles, as a marker of self-conscious social rebellion, Rastafarians resemble Hindu Sādhus, although Rastas do not believe in the need to relinquish all their belongings or to spend their lives in service at funerary rites. Nonetheless, dreadlocks are a statement of boldness, confidence, and self-realization, and they uphold biblical commandments against shaving. Dreadlocks emblematically express InI consciousness, and they (ideally) give voice to an experiential understanding of the inseparability of the self from "Jah."

Furthermore, "Dread talk," an in-group language that builds social cohesion, contains an abundance of "I" words. Terms such as "InI consciousness" signify an understanding of the presence of a divine positive energy in the world. So too "ital" suggests the importance of natural foods, and "irie" means to pick up positive feelings and vibrations. Drawing on an African legacy of imbuing words with intrinsic power, potency, vibration, and effective agency, dread talk is also a means of "chanting down" the social, political, and economic institutions of repression found in Babylon.[74] Here again we discover in the Rastafarian tradition a utopian tendency—for in that chanting down, they mean to fashion a new social order based on an individual form of freedom that simultaneously supports the commonweal.

As a result of repatriation projects in Africa, the Rastafarian movement now boasts of members in Ethiopia, Ghana, Malawi, Benin, and South Africa. Their spread through the Caribbean, Europe, the Americas, and to the farthest flung locations on the planet through the popularity of Reggae music continues, despite incisive and important criticisms concerning the role of women in Rastafarian societies. Even in light of what many see as serious shortcomings regarding gender equality (vis-à-vis a proclaimed doctrine of inclusiveness), the Rastafarian movement continues to grow, perhaps due to their compelling stories of exile from Africa, history of captivity in Jamaica, and longing for Zion. Certainly, the Rastafarian presence in Ethiopia predates the emergence of Reggae music as a tool for evangelizing,[75] and their unique form of "rude" audacity, social critique, and religious mysticism mixed with a veneration of the cannabis plant has captured the imagination of a certain segment of an unrepresented and disadvantaged global underclass.

By way of summary, let us reflect on the historical and cultural sweep of our spiritual survey of cannabis. So far, it has taken us from the ancient Indus Valley and Iranian Plateau, over the Tibetan Himalayas, and into China. We have traveled through the Middle East into Africa, and negotiated the murkiness of the remote past to arrive in the twenty-first century—all in order to follow a remarkable story of humankind's manifold relationship with a single plant. In the next chapter, we return to Abraham Maslow's theory of peak-experiences, because those moments of awakening are at the heart of religious experience and the harmonious functioning between body and mind. In order to emphasize their universalism across time and place, we next juxtapose two distinctive mystical traditions—one from the Old World, and the other from the New World.

5

PEAK-EXPERIENCES AND THE INEFFABLE

We began this investigation with the supposition that a wave of new laws permitting the use of marijuana as medicine in the United States, together with ongoing legalization and decriminalization efforts, are making the way clear for engagement with cannabis on a deeper level of physical and psychological healing. To support that assertion, we surveyed the manifold ways in which cannabis has been utilized medicinally, sacramentally, and recreationally throughout human history and noted the coevolution of that plant with human civilization.

In India, we identified Vedic soma rites that drove peak-experiences, the cannabis-inspired adoration of Shiva, the radical nondualism in the *Upanishads* and *Bhagavad Gītā*, and the influence of Ayurvedic medicine on Tibetan and Chinese healing arts. In Tibetan Buddhism, we discovered a mélange of Vedānta, Shaivite Hinduism, Bön beliefs, and an esoteric knowledge of medical plants and herbs used as part of religious observation. The Chinese *Book of Songs* demonstrated the centrality of hemp as a foodstuff and essential fiber for cloth, canvas, and rope. In Chinese pharmacopoeia, cannabis is deployed (like any healing herb) in the framework of an understanding of the integral connections between the body and the cosmos, the meridian system of channels and acupoints through which qi and blood circulate, and the relationship between mental integration and physical wellness.

On the Iranian plateau, we found cannabis-inspired Zoroastrian priests probing the religious experiences of Zarathustra, a Mithraic entheogenic Eucharist, as well as inward-looking Sufi mystics who snubbed religious prohibitions on intoxicants and pursued God in a hookah. We located evidence of hemp production in ancient Egypt, took note of the import of cannabis to Christian monastics training in Ethiopia and Egypt, and followed the dispersion of that plant across Africa with Islamic soldiers and merchants. Among dagga cults and tribes such as the Khoikhoi, Zulu, Pygmy, and Bena-Riamba, marijuana replaced native herbal ingredients in established medicinal formulas, provided a performance booster for laborious activities, and offered an important means of social cohesion. In the Caribbean, a group of renegade Rastafarians, yearning for a spiritual leader and anxious to find a healing balm for the nations, made cannabis central to their worship of Jah.

We undertook this far-ranging journey to better appreciate the prominence of cannabis in the cultural and religious history of humankind, and through that understanding to discover ways that the conscientious person currently living in a country, state, or region with progressive marijuana laws might tap its potential as an agent of mental, physical, and spiritual well-being. To establish cannabis as an entheogen and vehicle for expanded consciousness, we return to peak-experiences and the state of intense concentrated attention that drives them. These moments of exaltation engender psychological integration and clarify perception, and such mental limpidity has positive repercussions on the physical body. To explore these assertions, the universal human propensity for ecstasy as a therapeutic modality is examined below in two mystical religions separated by time, place, culture, and language.

What Abraham Maslow called "peak-experiences" are the mystical, transcendental, ecstatic, epiphanic, or salvific moments that constitute the bedrock of human religious experience. To miss them, and to participate in symbol and ritual only, is a grievous loss—for religion is a state of mind, and peak-experiences are the raw material out of which religious philosophies are wrenched. As a scientist, Maslow analyzed religious experiences in the same manner that a psychologist would approach any such phenomenon—as secularly, empirically, objectively, descriptively, and as humanistically as possible—so as to get at an essential truth. For this reason, his work on the subject endures, and today a new generation of scientists and psychologists are bringing innovative technologies to bear in the quest to understand human consciousness and religious experience.

A natural mystic who never took psychedelics, Maslow discovered that peak-experiences occur spontaneously in the lives of highly creative "self-actualizing" people (such as Albert Einstein and Eleanor Roosevelt), and that they provide "a deep sense of inner security and often constitute a source of strength during periods of suffering or struggle in life and as one approaches death."[1] Yet, many people who have such experiences often do not share them for fear of being misunderstood or viewed as eccentric or even mentally ill, but for Maslow they represented forays into the higher reaches of human nature. Even if unrecognized as religious experience, when peak-experiences occur, they "tend to be humbly received."[2]

Several weighty reasons compel the diligent pursuit of peak-experiences: the possibility of curing nonpathological psychoses and neuroses through them, the positive transformative potential they offer to all human beings, as well as the socially ameliorative consequences of those shifts in consciousness—a fact recognized thousands of years ago in China by ever-pragmatic Confucians and mystical Daoists alike. A great urgency exists for people to "wake up" to the necessity of grounding the self in reality, rather than in individualistic and collective egoic fantasies. If "we are the world," and become aware of it even momentarily through peak-experiences, then we must bear witness to the suffering wrought by remaining out of accord with reality. The violence that human beings inflict on the earth, not recognizing the earth as the sustainer of their life, is rivaled only by the brutality perpetrated on each other through social inequality, war, and prejudice (false "prejudgments") of all sorts.

Nonetheless, as more individuals learn to identify, cultivate, and prolong peak-experiences, we stand to witness considerable social betterment, given that human society is ultimately a set of relationships, the quality of which reflect our inner selves. Therefore when more of us become aware of "the temporal and the eternal realms of consciousness," then to resolve tensions and conflicts, we may choose the avenue for dialogue rather than belligerence. The increasing interest in yoga, meditative disciplines, world religions, and sacramental and therapeutic uses of entheogens augurs well for a peaceful evolution of our species.[3]

Maslow clearly recognized this transformational potential of peak-experiences, and he argued that they were not the exclusive province of institutionalized religion (which he found woefully out of touch with authentic spirituality). Sustained religious practice does not constitute the exclusive route to this central component of self-actualization. Maslow argued that sexual love, philosophical insight, athletic performance, having a child, or deep admiration of art were all potential triggers for peak-experiences.[4] Self-transcendent moments are not always recognized as a variety of mystical religious experience, yet if the fundamentally enlightened nature of consciousness is recognized, peak experiences can open the way to sustained awakening.

The thirteenth-century Japanese priest Dōgen Zenji reportedly counseled one student, who remained stubbornly oblivious to his own Buddha-nature (perhaps in the erroneous pursuit of a more "fantastical" or "visionary" state of consciousness): "Do not think you will necessarily be aware of your own enlightenment."[5] Likewise, the writer Eckhart Tolle initially failed to understand the enduring shift that took place when a deep depression, which left him in utter misery, suddenly abated one morning. Tolle comprehended that something changed in his consciousness, for his egoic "self-talk" decreased by 80 percent, and he could hear the birds chirping—whereas before there was mental noise, distraction, and self-inflicted suffering. By his own account, only after reading the works of mystics such as Laozi, Meister Eckhart, and Krishnamurti did he fully appreciate the transformation wrought in his consciousness as "awakening" or "enlightenment."[6]

In that recognition, Tolle noted his ability to rise above thought and abide in still presence, which manifested itself outwardly as a calm detachment and total surrender to the present moment. In the excerpt below, Tolle bemoans the failure of institutional religion to deliver genuine peak-experiences to large numbers of people, a point Maslow repeatedly asserts in *Religions, Values, and Peak-Experiences*:

> Since ancient times, spiritual masters of all traditions have pointed to the Now as the key to the spiritual dimension. Despite this, it seems to have remained a secret. It is certainly not taught in churches and temples. If you go to a church, you may hear readings from the Gospels such as "Take no thought for the morrow; for the morrow shall take thought for the things of itself," or "Nobody who puts his hands to the plow and *looks back* is fit for the Kingdom of God." Or you might hear the passage about the beautiful flowers that are not anxious about tomorrow but live with ease in the timeless Now and are provided for abundantly by God. The depth and radical nature of these teachings is

not recognized. No one seems to realize that they are meant to be lived and so bring about a profound inner transformation.

The whole essence of Zen consists in walking along the razor's edge of Now—to be so utterly, so completely *present* that no problem, no suffering, nothing that is not *who you are* in your essence, can survive in you. In the Now, in the absence of time, all your problems dissolve. Suffering needs time; it cannot survive in the Now.[7]

Tolle reminds us that the present moment, not the church tithe box, is the primary entryway into the here-now—and it confers all of the benefits that spring out of living authentically from the center of being.

One of the religious aspects of peak-experiences Maslow identified was the arising of "B-cognition" (or "Being cognition"), which is more passive, receptive, and humble than awareness of being. He found that "B-cognition" made people instinctively more object-centered (rather than self-oriented), and that its proper functioning in consciousness permitted people to perceive their surroundings in a more consequential manner.[8] Moreover, the unitive consciousness that accompanies B-cognition removes selfhoods that obscure a clear perception of prodigious beauty in the world. As noted earlier, Maslow discovered that peak-experiences occur in every time period, culture, religious tradition, economic class, and gender (irrespective of localisms), and they constitute a core human experience and exemplify a form of religious revelation that has played a pivotal role in the history of religion.[9]

However, Maslow argues that some people are naturally more open to self-transcendence than others, and the mystical experiences of "peakers" can hardly be shared with "nonpeakers" (hence their ineffability). In spite of that limitation of language, peak-experiences are relatable to other "peakers" and discernible as a pattern or cluster of religious experiences. For mystically inclined individuals, the buildings, rituals, dogmas, specialized personnel, and ceremonials that accompany institutional religious practice become secondary to transcendental experience. Profoundly authentic religious persons might adopt the outward forms of religion, but such inner cognition is the ground of peak-experience.

"Nonpeakers" represent a form of religious expression closely associated with the legalistic organizational personality. This legalistic-ecclesiastic—or the conservative "organization man"—is the officer who is loyal to the bureaucratic structures built up around the original revelation of a religious leader (whether Zoroaster, Siddhārtha Gautama, Jesus of

Nazareth, or Muhammad). In contrast to the firsthand religious experiences of these and other mystics, the personality structure of "nonpeakers" causes them to be extremely (or completely) rational and materialistic, and they fear letting go of their logically organized knowledge. So great is the chasm between these two personality types that Maslow supposes organized religion may sometimes actually be the opponent of authentic religious experience. [10] If he overstates the case, it is not without making an important point: religion devoid of experiential understanding means reducing a living truth to an empty ritual, the finger and not the moon, the note but not the song.

In their most positive form, organized religions may be regarded as the result of an effort to communicate peak-experiences to "nonpeakers." A grave danger exists, however, when those holding influential positions in religious organizations are no longer directly connected to the spiritual experiences of their traditions' founders—and instead concretize (or venerate) religious symbols. [11] "Idolatry," the worship of the outward symbolic representations of a religion, stands in stark contrast to the cultivation of the transcendental experiences upon which they were established. Scripture not only springs out of a desire to preserve important cultural histories, but a need to point the way toward authentic spirituality. Religious orthodoxy threatens to strip the world of sacredness—when its symbols are revered with no firsthand understanding of the mystical experiences that inform them.

Because Maslow published *Religions, Values, and Peak-Experiences* in 1964, during the antiestablishment counterculture movements in the West, some readers may wonder what he thought about employing organic and chemical substances to stimulate self-transcendent experiences, particularly in "nonpeakers." While he does not address cannabis directly, as he considered it a mildly psychoactive plant, Maslow sounds a cautious note concerning the use of stronger entheogens to elicit peak-experiences. Writing three years before the "Summer of Love" in the Haight-Ashbury neighborhood of San Francisco (but ten years after the publication of Aldous Huxley's *Doors of Perception*), Maslow agreed that psilocybin, mescaline, and LSD might produce peak-experiences in some individuals under the proper circumstances, and he thereby left open the possibility that they might be employed to bridge the chasm between more mystically minded "peakers" and those caught more firmly in the grip of egoic thinking and institutional imperatives.

In point of fact, recent double-blind research studies at the Johns Hopkins University indicate that many positive outcomes result from psilocybin taken in safe clinical environments. In controlled settings, attendant physicians act to alleviate any anxiety attending the onset of the entheogens by reassuring patients of the safety of the experiment and guiding their "trips" with music, contemplation, and discussion. The people who seem to benefit most from psychedelic courses of treatment include those suffering from post-traumatic stress disorder, chronic addictive tendencies, and cancer. For patients facing terminal illnesses, psychedelic regimes assist in awakening a greater acceptance of human mortality by providing access to the transcendence of time and space (as ordinarily experienced), bestowing a sense of blessedness, and stimulating feelings of unity with the universe. Researchers at Johns Hopkins found that all participants in whom peak-experiences were elicited, including novices and experienced meditators, gained a heightened sense of personal well-being generally accompanied by altruistic feelings toward others, greater aesthetic appreciation, increased sensitivity and creative thinking, and a broad-minded tolerance of others' viewpoints and values. [12]

In previous chapters, we outlined a cultural history of intentional use of marijuana as a vehicle for peak-experiences, and the self-transformations with which they are associated. As should be evident from that investigation, the milder and gentler cannabis plant offers access to many of the therapeutic benefits of stronger entheogens, most notably when combined with concentrated activities (such as meditation, contemplative prayer, chanting, or other such exercises) to actualize self-transcendence. Maslow demonstrated that peak-experiences are universally observable in societies, cultures, and religious traditions around the world. To illustrate that point, the remainder of this chapter juxtaposes Mediterranean Mystery cults and Native American shamanism as evidence of the enduring importance of peak-experiences for enhancing perception, achieving self-actualization, and effecting social amelioration.

Unitive consciousness, Maslow observes, is always a possibility for thoughtful individuals ("peakers" and "nonpeakers" alike)—and most of us have had, or are capable of having, peak-experiences. [13] Half of all Americans report experiencing sudden and often fleeting shifts in perception associated with self-transcendent experiences, and in their most positive inflections, they embed an alternate set of "B-values" (associated with B-cognition) in the personality, including: uprightness, simplicity, self-sufficiency, wholeness, and the transcendence of dichotomy (duality). They also instill in people a strong sense of justice and fairness and result in greater acceptance of life circumstances. Individuals who embody B-values are "self-actualizers" because they possess a clear perception of reality, make good judgments, accept shortcomings in themselves and others, value independent freedom from outside authorities, enjoy a sense of fellowship with humanity, and tend to prefer solitude.[14] Enduring transformations of the self often follow such peak moments of clarity, harmony, and bliss—and they infuse the world with meaning and fill it with light.

For this reason, peak-experiences arguably foreshadow a new stage in human evolution (one that will be more psychological than physiological), as the universe becomes self-aware through the capacity of the awakened human mind to witness the ongoing act of creation. This understanding is beautifully summarized in the opening lines of Alan Watts's *Art of Contemplation*:

> The individual is an aperture through which the whole energy of the universe is aware of itself, a vortex of vibrations in which it realizes itself as man or beast, flower or star—not alone, but as central to all that surrounds it. These centers are not, as may seem, apart from their surroundings, but stand in mutual relationship to them—center to circumference—in the same way as the magnetic poles. It is thus that each center anywhere implies all other centers elsewhere. The individual is not, therefore, only a center. He is the entire surround centered at this time or this place.[15]

Historically speaking, people have been "waking up" to this new mode of nondualistic perception for thousands of years, and they were often labeled prophets, seers, or even sometimes heretics. As this evolution in human consciousness speeds up, brief and sustained peak-experiences will become more commonplace. It appears, concludes William A. Richards, that our species "could well be moving toward a more peaceful world utopia of some kind."[16]

In the ancient Greco-Roman Mediterranean world, one way that people fostered peak-experiences was through initiation into one of several Mystery traditions, all of which offered important alternatives to state-sponsored religions. Prior to the arrival of Christianity, religious worship meant petitioning invisible supernatural beings believed responsible for harvests, natural disasters, health and prosperity, and even the prospects for victory or loss in battle. Every community in the Greco-Roman world acted as its own religious authority, and as a result there existed a good deal of variation in terms of devout expressions and ritual obligations. Some of the most commonplace customs included prayer offerings to major deities, as well as the observance of festivals in their honor. Dramatic performances and religious processions included animal sacrifices, but they created a nexus through which the gods would commune with their worshippers over sanctified meals. Small cults carried their shrines and statues from place to place, while larger organizations had buildings in which to house cult sculptures.[17] While not generally discernible to human beings, the intentions of the gods might nevertheless be divined by reading the entrails of sacrificial animals, consulting the stars, or interpreting omens in the environment.

Inhabitants of the Greco-Roman world participated in Mystery religion ceremonies by the thousands—and these events were meant to culminate in ecstatic peak-experiences. Attendees underwent ritual purifications, wore charmed amulets, and made offerings at shrines to ward off malevolent influences. Mystery cults, generally speaking, draw from a mixture of traditions (including Orientalism), but are most often associated with Demeter (goddess of the harvest), Dionysus (god of wine and theater), and Mithras (i.e., Mithra, god of justice and contractual truth). These and other mystery religions insisted on secrecy, although they offered knowledge concealed from the general public in return. Inductees handled revered objects and were taught their symbolic meanings, and they sometimes partook of ceremonial meals. Mystery rites reached an apex in collective moments of heightened perception, at the centers of which were symbolic death and resurrection. The Mysteries of Isis, for instance, required the "voluntary death" of neophytes as a prerequisite to spiritual rebirth. Likewise, initiates in the Mysteries of Cybele were viewed as occupying a state of dying that foreshadowed promised renewal.[18] The *Mithras Liturgy* included some elements of rebirth, too.

The most revered of all cults were the Eleusinian Mysteries; celebrated every autumn at Eleusis in the Attic countryside outside of Athens. For more than one thousand years, men and women once thronged to witness the rites or be initiated into them. At their heart, a mythical account of the changing seasons upon which human agricultural production depended. Penned in the fifth or sixth century BCE (and attributed to Homer), the

Hymns to Demeter recount the abduction of Persephone by Hades, and they were performed for the duration of the eight-day festival held during the autumn sowing.[19] Unbeknownst to Demeter, Hades, the god of the underworld, secures prior consent to abduct her daughter Persephone—and make her his consort. Furious at Zeus for permitting such a violent act against their daughter, Demeter wanders the earth until she arrives at Eleusis. There, she discloses her divine identity to the inhabitants of the town, prevents the grain from growing, and demands that a temple be erected in her honor. After its completion, she reveals the rites that the populace must perform to appease her anger.

Demeter's strategy is shrewd, for before long it deprives the other gods of their sacrifices, and it ensures that they face starvation along with the mortals. Seeking a quick solution to this standoff, Zeus orders Demeter back to Mount Olympus. Still livid, the goddess demands the return of their daughter Persephone as the sole price for her mollification. Zeus relents and commands Hades to release the young woman. The god of the underworld complies, but not before placing a pomegranate seed in the young woman's mouth. Having partaken of that single morsel from the underworld, Persephone is obliged to return and spend three months of every year with Hades. During that fallow period, grain does not grow.

Finding their final form somewhere around the fifth century BCE, the Eleusinian Mysteries continued until the fourth or fifth century (after which time Christianity reigned supreme in the region). The ruins of the sanctuary at Eleusis contain vestiges of a small number of buildings surrounded by a wall. Conspicuously lacking, in comparison to sanctuaries for comparable gods and goddesses, was a grand temple for Demeter. Cult activities at Eleusis took place outside around open-air altars far removed from the sanctuary proper (and sacrificial offerings were not normally made inside the compound). The Hall of Mysteries, a large square building supported by columns where the dramatic and most secretive part of the rituals took place, included steps around the perimeter upon which participants and spectators sat or stood. At its largest, after centuries of expansion, the Hall of Mysteries held nearly three thousand people.[20]

Inductees participated in the Eleusinian Mysteries for two years (divided into the Lesser Mysteries and the Greater Mysteries). During nocturnal events, ritual participators experienced terror and pain in order to gain personal knowledge of the agonies endured by Persephone and Demeter. Mythic reenactments gave everyone in attendance an opportunity to acknowledge the power of the seasons to proffer or withhold a fertile harvest—and to express appropriate gratitude and humility. The mysteries featured multiple attempts to induce spiritual rapture through fasting, ritual ordeal, and the ceremonial ingestion of plant substances. The enforcement of cult codes of secrecy, combined with the passage of time, make it hard to reconstruct what took place during clandestine Mystery rites, but they seem to have involved going hungry prior to drinking *kykeon*—an aqueous blend of barley grouts, fleabane, and other plant compounds (including a grassy weed called darnel or tares that was subject to ergot infestation).[21] *Kykeon* was highly psychoactive, and at the Eleusinian liturgy, ritual dramatics reached a highpoint in concert with its ingestion.

Most probably, the nighttime revelries of the Mysteries focused around dramatic reenactments of the rape of Persephone and her subsequent return to the world of the living. As part of orchestrated performances, second-year initiates (and those returning after formal induction) might glimpse Persephone sitting forlorn in a rock hollow in the underworld, or conversely witness her happy reunion with Demeter.[22] A fragment from a lost work by Plutarch provides a sense of how that climatic scene at the Eleusinian Mystery might have looked. He describes a process of induction that resembles those found in other mystery traditions: initiates trotting frightening paths in darkness until, shivering and sweating, panic filled and bewildered, they find their way to open meadows where dances, music, and hallowed recitations took place. It was a holy vision following terrifying experiences with the "underworld."

Mystery Cults worked at the intersection of religious intoxication and peak-experience—and they represent a significant attempt by human beings to reach the divine by all means necessary. In this respect, the Eleusinian Mysteries echo Vedic soma rites and Zoroastrian *haoma* rituals, in so far as they esteem religion a living force that must be experienced directly—and not something abstract, symbolic, or representational. The ingestion of entheogens, such as *kykeon*, at Eleusis occurred annually, and only in sacramental contexts. Breaking the Eleusinian rites into paired sequences signaled that (plant-induced) ecstatic experiences ought to be contemplated for a year before returning to them, so that worshippers might incorporate the spiritual lessons learned from them into their daily lives. In fact, use of *kykeon* in secular settings and outside of parameters established by tradition, earned one the wrath of the general public. Such was the case with Alcibiades who stood accused of profaning the Mysteries when he served that psychoactive beverage for recreational purposes in his residence and allegedly revealed secret rites. (In chapter 6, we consider how the indiscriminate use of psychedelics contributed to the descent of hippie subculture into decadence during the 1960s and 1970s).

Imported by merchants from Scythia or possibly India, cannabis was used extensively in human medicine and animal husbandry in the ancient Greco-Roman world. Botanical and medical writers such as Dioscorides, Galen, and Oribasius underscored the pharmacological features of the cannabis plant.[23] In his *Natural History*, Pliny the Elder wrote that the juice of cannabis seeds extracted worms or insects from the ears,[24] and he recorded that it was good for the stomachs of cattle, treating burns topically, and lessening the pain of arthritis and gout. In the second century, the physician Galen noted the virtues of hemp-cakes for establishing and maintaining well-being.[25] Accounts from the celebrations of the mystery religions, as well as in epic poetry, show that many other psychoactive plants (including opium, hemp, psilocybin mushrooms, darnel, and the fungal parasite ergot) found places in ancient medical traditions and spiritual rites.[26]

The most conspicuous cannabis enthusiasts in the Greco-Roman world, however, were the Scythians. A seminomadic central Asian tribe encountered by the Greek historian Herodotus during his travels in the fifth century BCE, the Scythians congregated along the Black Sea and spoke a variety of Indo-Iranian dialects. An Iranian people with a reputation for barbarity, they were relatively tall (with men often reaching six feet) and wore long braided tunics trimmed with fur and leather. The immense steppe east of the Danube River, over which they roamed, linked Europe with Asia. Mounted on horseback, the Scythians were highly mobile for the day, and ample grasslands made ideal pastures (that required almost no human labor to maintain) for cattle, sheep, and horses.

We know little about the dress habits of women because they were less often depicted in surviving artifacts, combined with the fact that organic materials do not preserve well. However, it appears that upper-class Scythian women donned long robes replete with gold ornamentation, leather boots, and elaborate headdresses (at least on ceremonial occasions). Less affluent Scythian womenfolk worked at planting wheat, rye, flaxseed, hemp, peas, and other essential crops, and must have contented themselves with simpler attire. The Scythians traded goods with neighboring groups, including the Greeks, for necessities and coveted luxury items—and the Scythian love of Greek wine is still legendary. Men and women were equally keen devotees of all things Dionysian, as wine collections and drinking vessels found in the graves of wealthy women attest.

Herodotus reported that funeral ceremonies for prominent members of the Scythian community included ritual purging. Afterward, as was the custom of this particular group of Scythians (whom the Greek historian met near modern-day Bulgaria), mourners sat in a "sweat lodge" excavated in the earth and covered with woolen mats. Inside, bronze cauldrons held hot rocks that created a sauna-like environment. Seed-laden hemp flowers (stored in leather bags) were cast onto the scorching stones to make a cannabis vapor bath. [27] The combined effect of the heat and cannabis steam was one of salutary healing in a time of sorrow and contemplation of death. The Scythians left behind evidence of six-pole tents that could be erected quickly as portable cannabis vapor baths. [28] However, it remains unclear whether marijuana was utilized for purely ritualistic purposes, or whether it was a more common part of everyday Scythian life. Whichever the case, archeologists have unearthed graves of Scythian men and women that contained working apparatuses for inhaling cannabis. [29]

The countless burial mounds that dot Eastern Europe rank among the most enduring artifacts of Scythian civilization. When constructed for a king or prince, a royal tomb might require the excavation of more than fourteen thousand cubic feet of soil to form the underground chamber. After the formal funerary rites were held, the shaft of the tomb was filled in, leaving the burial chamber, where the body rested, open. Over the filled-in shaft, rocks and soil were piled to form a mound that could reach sixty or seventy feet in height. [30] Raising such mounds required concerted community effort, and once completed, sacrifices were offered at their base, followed by a memorial feast.

Surviving gold work by Scythian artisans illustrates the centrality of war, hunting, and animal husbandry to their everyday lives. In scenes of gold, Scythian men wear lengthy beards with long, flowing hair. In battle, and during hoarding raids, they dressed in dazzling armor and made a fearsome sight mounted on their steeds with their crossbows, long swords, lances, and axes. Unlike their female Greek counterparts, Scythian women participated in battle (at least after uniting with a nearby tribe of Amazon warriors). Female combatants were buried with their weapons, and their remains offer evidence of the injuries that they sustained while fighting.[31] Scythian women also contributed to hunting parties, rode horses, and took part in the martial games that constituted part of their leisure time activities. These martial exploits of the Scythians helped to create an empire that endured for several hundred years.

With the decline and disappearance of the Scythians, we depart the ancient world for good, and turn instead to Native American shamanism, peak-experience, and the ineffable. As we have seen in previous encounters with shamanism in the Indus Valley, on the Iranian Plateau, and in Tibet, peak-experiences encourage healing of the mind and body, but they are also "ineffable." The difficulty of communicating transcendent states of consciousness resembles the challenge of trying to describe the thrill of a bungee dive or parachute jump to a "nonjumper." Try as she might, the adventurer struggles to find words adequate to that task and eventually resorts to comparison, simile, and metaphor to convey the core experience of the jump. Ultimately, though, to really know what it is like, one has no choice but to dive. Short of that, one's understanding of bungee jumping remains merely intellectual and conceptual.

The term "ineffable" denotes the quality or state of things incapable of being expressed in language. In religious studies, the deployment of ineffability is generally limited to mystical experiences, since the object of contemplation is undifferentiated and possesses no qualities that can be represented or communicated except paradoxically.[32] Keeping this important feature of ineffability in mind, let us briefly consider several core shamanistic beliefs held among Native American tribes on both continents in order to shed further light on the universality of peak-experiences, and their unique expressions based on the time, place, and social context of their unfolding.

Ecstasy is the central practice of the shaman, and magicians, sorcerers, medicine women, and ecstatic healers are found in indigenous societies around the globe and throughout the entire history of religion.[33] While terms such as "magician" and "sorcerer" may sound archaic to some contemporary readers, or, even worse, suggest occult activities, in their own communities shamans are credited with an ability to cure mental and physical illnesses and perform miracles. They generate ecstasy, the touchstone of religious experience, and marshal this modality of healing by practicing a variety of techniques for cultivating bliss. [34] In the parlance of Judeo-Christianity, shamans are among the "elect," since they have privileged access to a region of the sacred unavailable to other members of their communities. The intensity of their religious experience frequently sets shamans apart from a young age as a spiritual adept (as is also the case with many saints and mystics).

Among Native American tribes, shamans may assume hereditary positions, but the sheer fierceness of an individuals' spirituality also justifies entry into that highly esteemed vocation. Many American shamans specialize in the art of the trance, during which the soul leaves the body and ascends upward into the heavens or downward to the underworld. In such visionary realms, shamans cultivate and maintain relationships with the spirit world (where souls of dead persons, nature spirits, and animal spirits rove), and they seek therein possession by those forces, or preferably control over them. [35] Shamans encountering divine or semidivine beings in trances or dream states may query them regarding the causes of illness or misfortune. The shaman likewise prays and petitions guardian spirits for protection, knowledge, or supplementary powers—feats that sometimes require learning secret animal languages. For instance, one Nicola Valley shaman acquired a "coyote language" during his vision quest, and he later used it in healing incantations. [36]

Shamans in North America draw power from an assortment of divine beings: the ancestral souls of deceased shamans, mythical animals, as well as certain sacred objects and cosmic zones. An augmentation of shamanistic powers occurs spontaneously, after deliberate questing, or by way of initiatory ordeals usually considered necessary to make such acquisitions meaningful. Native American shamans on vision quest retreat to caves or similarly austere spaces to pursue visions by way of prolonged intense concentrated activities. If dream visions do not come quickly enough, then adepts perform rigorous ritual purifications until guardian spirits may be discerned, engaged, and learned from. [37] Among North American Plains Indian societies, vision questing for protector spirits constitutes a kind of culturally prescribed dream, hallucination, or unusual auditory or visual experience that is interpreted as coming from supernatural entities and results in the acquisition of power, advice, or ritual privileges. [38]

For this reason, the symbolic content of shamanistic visions tends to conform to existing cultural belief systems, which validates their form, substance, and behavioral directives. Some North American shamans even proclaimed the spiritual regeneration of entire communities using the power that they acquired during tribulations related to their vision quests. Religious practices such as these endure today, but they were particularly important to maintaining community—a cohesion in the wake of the disease and genocide that accompanied European settlement of the Americas. A similar ganja "vision quest" exists in Jamaica among the working poor (where seeing images of little dancing women or men of different colors marks a kind of rite of passage to adulthood and validates the smoker's status within the peer group).[39]

Native American shamans, who acquire knowledge through direct experience with the supernatural world, use it for the positive function of healing—or for less gallant ends as sorcerers. Some mystical shamanist sects in North America, such as the Ghost Dance religions, employ séance to determine the cause of disease, expel pathogenic substances creating illness, or locate a lost soul in order to restore a person's life force.[40] Like the Mediterranean Mystery traditions, Native American shamanistic initiations are shrouded in secret rites, but they might involve a candidate's symbolic death and resurrection, ecstatic visits to lands of the Dead or Sky, the insertion of magical substances into the initiate's body, the revelation of clandestine doctrines, and instruction in techniques of curative healing.[41] All of these initiatory ordeals help to bring about mental transformation, but they also represent therapeutic approaches used to discover and remove the source of illness—and to bolster the wellness of the body and mind.

In some regions of the South American continent, shamans turn the souls of the newly dead into intermediaries between human beings and the spirit world. Shamans also perform important rituals, defend the tribe from malevolent spirits, facilitate births, reveal future events, and identify fruitful hunting spots. They are credited with the ability to perform marvels, such as magical flight and swallowing hot coals. As fantastic as those aptitudes seem, the magico-religious potency of shamans provides the basis for their social authority. For instance, South American shamans undertake celestial visitations to petition spirits on behalf of an entire community and learn sacred songs from birds and other animals, as well. They recognize the medicinal virtues of plants and other substances and adapt that understanding to a variety of healing techniques, including: fumigation, song, body massage, trance, and the removal of pathogenic substances by way of suction.[42] These and other shamanistic healing techniques alter the consciousness of practitioners and their patients in ways considered positive (in that they evoke new ways of knowing and being in the world). Their activities in the spirit realm also bestow upon shamans the enhanced cognitive capabilities associated with more actualized modes of psychological integration.

The correspondences among shamanistic practices around the world, not just those in North and South America, point to an innate and universal propensity for peak-experiences in human consciousness. Syncopated movement, chanting, praying, drumming, fasting, abstaining from sexual acts, and ceremonial rites all evoke ecstatic states of consciousness—as do other practices: the ingestion of psychoactive substances, undergoing sensory and social deprivation, and dream incubation. The resulting euphoric states mark entryway into the spirit world, and they allow contact with ancestors and other supernatural beings, as well as the acquisition of mystical powers during soul journeys.[43] By bolstering the social unity needed to overcome stresses on their resources and challenges by competing groups, South American shamans contributed to the fitness and continuance of their communities. In addition, they fostered their community's adaptive potential by encouraging the reduced ego-centeredness among its members that comes with strengthened solidarity. In this respect, we might also regard shamanism as an evolutionary survival mechanism.

Among some Native American peoples there persists a belief in a medicine path operating at the matrix of religious practice, shamanistic ecstasy, herbal remedies, peak-experiences, and spiritual healing. Collectively, Roger Walsh calls these and other devices humankind's first "technology of transcendence," through which poured the sacred visions that sustained indigenous communities. Historically speaking, the ritual use of psychedelics among native tribes in North and South America received extremely short shrift from anthropologists until the 1970s, when interest grew in consuming plant substances (including peyote, ayahuasca, and a variety of mushrooms) as a means of better understanding the religious worldviews and shamanistic practices of the people whom they were studying.[44]

A relative latecomer to the New World, cannabis arrived with the African victims of the European slave trade in the sixteenth century and quickly spread throughout both continents. In the highland terrain they inhabited in Mexico, Tepehuán people grew corn and other stable foods on little plots of land, practiced traditional handicrafts such as weaving, and herded small animals (with goats providing a source of meat, milk, and cheese). Sometime during the sixteenth century, Jesuit missionaries appeared, and by the early part of the next century a messianic figure named Quautlatas rose up to resist Spanish domination of the region, albeit unsuccessfully. Baptized as a Christian, he rallied his people around the image of a broken cross, struck at colonial holdings, killed Spanish sympathizers, and ended the silver mining that desecrated the natural landscape.[45]

In cannabis, the Tepehuán Indians discovered an occasional substitute for the peyote that they collected for sacrosanct ceremonies.[46] Bestowing on the plant the sobriquet "Sacred Rose," they attributed to marijuana the ability to stimulate loquaciousness, enhance social interaction, and serve as a gateway to religious experiences. In some of their rituals (which blended aboriginal beliefs with Christian symbolism), the Tepehuán placed the contents of bundles of paper on an altar. The Sacred Rose would rest there, surrounded by small bells, incense holders, and whistles that served as objects of attention for attendants who made daily offerings or provided ceremonial water refreshments. The men and women associated with the altar were especially privileged, since their positions permitted the regular consumption of the Sacred Rose. From that advantageous station, they derived social statures equal to their special relationship with the supernatural world.

During Sacred Rose ceremonies, guests of the priests, who tended the consecrated cannabis plants, participated in its ritualistic ingestion during occasions featuring music and worship. As the Tepehuán musicians played on, inspired by the marijuana that they consumed, priestesses danced and priests purified members of the community by tapping branches of that hallowed plant on their shoulders. Candles were lit, and whistles and bells announced the arrival of the spirits. Thereafter, the notes that the musicians played were considered those of the Sacred Rose. Everyone in attendance hummed along with melodic lyrical phrases like:

> Today, we who have taken it
> shout with joy
> today we have seen
> and we who are taking it
> we are rejoicing.[47]

For the Tepehuán people, cannabis epitomized the living impulse of the universe—as if it were "a small piece of the heart of God."[48]

Competing with stronger entheogens, including peyote and mescaline, cannabis did not always arrive at the center of religious rites in the Americas, although the Cuna Indians of Panama were known to smoke marijuana communally in tribal meetings, and the Cora Indians in the Sierra Madre Occidental turned to it when indigenous plant herbs became unavailable.[49] Much farther north and east, the Iroquois people smoked tobacco mixed with herbs, and their pharmacopoeia included cannabis, along with plants like datura (jimsonweed). Most Iroquois medicinal plants were collected and harvested to treat symptoms of illness such as fever, weakness, chills, and vomiting.[50] Indian hemp dogbane may have been used as a blood purifier and laxative, but cannabis was believed to speed recovery, particularly in patients reluctant to acknowledge their own wellness.[51] Since shamans attributed the effects of plants to their spirits, and not their chemical compositions, whole classes of florae were used in a variety of divinatory contexts.

This comprehensive knowledge of botanicals in Native American shamanistic medicine combined with an understanding that psychological anxiety, fear, and stress have negative effects on the body. Ritual treatments by respected shamans assist in reducing the physical manifestations of egoic thought and thereby hasten recovery. The earliest European observers of the Oneida and other Iroquois tribes in North America, for instance, took note of their employment of curing groups in which a dozen or so men danced around a patient while a woman chanted and rhythmically shook a rattle. Male shamans wore headbands, painted their faces red, threw or ate fire, and sucked objects out of the bodies of their patients.[52] The Oneida Iroquois honored dreams as well, and their shamans went to great pains to interpret them.

By way of summary, the juxtaposition of ancient Greco-Roman Mysteries with shamanistic practices of the Native American peoples lends credence to Maslow's assertion that religious peak-experiences are universal and perennial. While smoking herbs is a longstanding Native American practice, and one that early Europeans noted with interest,[53] regrettably the plants burned in "peace pipes" did little to reveal European duplicity toward Native Americans, or to enlighten white settlers, who were more intent on grabbing land than finding peak-experiences. Nonetheless, the ecstatic elements in indigenous shamanism have clear correlates in the use of entheogens and ceremonial rituals in the Mystery religions; they also affirm that the intentional use of psychoactive plants such as cannabis to stimulate the positive alteration of consciousness through peak-experiences may offer greater psychological integration and sense of well-being to serious-minded seekers.

6

HASHISH EATERS, HOBBITS' LEAF, AND THE PANTAGRUELION

In coming to the end of our historical survey, we turn to Europe, where at the beginning of the Renaissance cannabis helped to sustain the colonial enterprise by providing an important raw material for the rigging and sails that propelled the maritime vessels exploring Africa, Asia, and the New World. Along with new avenues for international trade opened by European merchants came an influx of new ideas. The term "renaissance" suggests cultural revitalization, and this was a European era when economic growth combined with a tidal wave of challenging thought from the fourteenth century to the seventeenth century (encouraged by the recovery of a Greco-Roman heritage). Jointly these trends drove a secular impulse for the rational and empirical investigation of the physical world, including the human body, and that pursuit permanently refigured the trajectory of Western civilization.

By the sixteenth century, European scholars had grappled for hundreds of years with the difficulty of synthesizing Christian salvation (and a belief in an afterlife) with Aristotelian science, materialistic philosophy, classical literature, and the new learning (i.e., humanism). Writers and intellectuals like Francesco Petrarca (Petrarch) and Giovanni Boccaccio helped to hasten that ideological move away from Church doctrine toward wider exploration and a spirit of free-inquiry.[1] They combed Church libraries and monasteries across the Italian peninsula for surviving fragments of classical texts authored by Cicero, Virgil, Horace, Livy, Plato, and Homer. Their efforts were aided by the fall of Baghdad to the

Mongols centuries earlier, which effectively brought the Islamic Renaissance to an end. In that legendary Middle Eastern city, thirty-six libraries preserved and augmented Greco-Roman classical learning, and that inflow of new material in the fields of medicine, science and technology, philosophy and religion, history, and law provided the impetus for a European revival.[2] The shift in emphasis from God to humankind resulted in an overall intensification of nationalism, skepticism, and secularism in Europe, as well.

François Rabelais, a Franciscan renunciate turned Benedictine monk, joined Desiderius Erasmus in his efforts to enrich Christianity by translating a classical literary heritage once largely lost to the Europeans. Inspired by his devotion to the new learning, and the broad-mindedness of the Renaissance more generally, Rabelais penned transgressive fictional narratives (some featuring cannabis) that were deemed such an outrageous assault on the staid status quo that more than once he fled persecution in fear for his life. Born into a well-to-do family in Touraine, Rabelais turned a happy childhood into an opportunity to read widely in literature and the sciences. As a young adult, he studied medicine and the law, but because his superiors in the order of St. Francis disapproved of his study of Greek (the language of a pagan religion), he was legally transferred from the Franciscans to the Benedictines. Eventually becoming a medical doctor and secular priest, Rabelais put his humanism into practice (and his life in jeopardy) by treating patients during the plague.[3]

In his bawdy and audacious novel *Gargantua and Pantagruel* (released sequentially over a thirty-year period), Rabelais combined vulgar humor with prodigious erudition and a piercing wit. That enormously clever serial work secured for Rabelais some formidable allies (who enjoyed his mockery of their dearest beliefs), but it also earned him the ire of powerful enemies in the Vatican and the Sorbonne. Although forced to escape to Italy in 1535 while writing *Gargantua*, and again about a decade later following the release of the third book, attempts to suppress the fourth book proved unsuccessful. The official censors greeted the release of each of the five books with impotent condemnation. For instance, the Council of Trent's *Index of Forbidden Books* in 1562 included *Gargantua and Pantagruel*—and it bestowed upon the unabashed Rabelais the ominous designation of "heretic of the first-class."[4] Despite this compellation, his fiction continued to find its way into publication, and he was read widely, if sometimes surreptitiously.

A virtuoso of all things scatological, Rabelais was one of the first European writers to draw attention to the psychoactive properties of cannabis. Although the five books of *Gargantua and Pantagruel* defy easy summation, they chronicle the lives of two fictional giants: Gargantua and his son Pantagruel. The first book to be written (although second in the series), *Pantagruel* amusingly satires chivalric tales and uninformed interpretations of scripture, and it pokes fun at many contemporaneous institutions of power. In the second book, the letter from Gargantua to his son Pantagruel "studying" in Paris ridicules the narrow scholasticism of the day and applauds a renewed enthusiasm for ancient learning. *Gargantua*, the first book, recounts how after an eleven-month pregnancy, Pantagruel came thundering into existence not with a whimper or cry, but with a loud and clear invitation to "Come drink, drink, drink!"[5] Befitting such an entry into the world, his parents baptized him with a long draught of wine.

The enormous appetite of the infant giant required the milk of 17,913 cows to quell, and as he grew, Pantagruel became fascinated with his own feces—a captivation that presented a considerable challenge in keeping the child clean.[6] In dealing with copious amounts of excrement, the natural outcome of his insatiable hunger and size, Pantagruel learned to become the greatest "arse-wiper" in the world—cleaning his bum on anything from a lady's lace bonnet, a March cat, his mother's gloves, the "linen sheets, on a blanket, the curtains, a cushion, a carpet, a baize tablecloth, a table napkin,"[7] and so on. Mercifully, Pantagruel eventually outgrew that feculent fascination with his own filth, and despite being driven nearly mad by Latin theologians in grammar school, he strove onward to gain a higher education. Still an uncouth and impetuous young man when he arrives in Paris, he steals bells from a prominent church to decorate his giant horse and participates in a battle to save abbey vineyards from an angry group of Paris bakers. A passionate wine enthusiast from birth, Gargantua rewards Friar John (Frère Jean) for helping him to defend that essential part of church property by founding the Abbey of Thélème in his honor.

The chapters dedicated to the Abbey of Thélème in *Gargantua* outline an ideal religious community, and his celebration of the herb pantagruelion in the third book anticipates secular and scientific engagements with cannabis on the continent. Trained in the mendicant Franciscan and monastic Benedictine traditions, Rabelais observed many abuses of power in the Catholic Church (abuses that motivated the Protestant Reformation). He also witnessed the decadence found in many Renaissance cloisters, and his Abbey of Thélème signals a critical attitude toward the monks, nuns, clerics, and scholars who inhabited them. He condemns their idleness, gluttony, lechery, venality, ignorance, mumbling of prayers, and general social uselessness.[8] Interestingly, the Rule of St. Benedict of Nursia and the Rule of St. Francis of Assisi separately addressed all of these depravities.

Not content to simply satirize Christian monastic orders and deride the entrenched corruptions of his day, Rabelais offered readers a fictional exemplar of a more authentically spiritual way of living communally. Gargantua, for instance, builds several unusual features into the Abbey of Thélème—but Frère Jean, in whose honor that religious complex is erected, is a mighty peculiar fellow. Frère Jean easily succumbs to gluttony, but he exhibits a merry disposition and straightforwardness that makes him jolly good company. In compensation for his numerous vices, he faithfully defends the oppressed, comforts the afflicted, succors the ailing, and stands watch over the abbey. In this sense, Frère Jean embodies the essence of "Pantagruelism," a certain lightness of spirit that lends itself to human conviviality and gives expression to a mode of living based on the humanist ideals of tolerance and empathy (that make communal living workable).

Unlike the typical Renaissance cloister, no walls surrounded the Abbey of Thélème. Hexagonal, with round towers at each of its corners, the abbey was six stories in height, constructed of stone, and decorated with gold work. A river ran along its north side, and on an ascent nearby stood a gateway, inscribed in antique lettering, which made clear that the Abbey of Thélème was a fortress of truth standing constant vigil in a world filled with duplicity, cunning, and selfishness. No hypocrites or bigots could enter Thélème; tightfisted lawyers and torturous canonists were similarly banned along with usurers, pandering scribes, and those filled with jealousy or envy. Only individuals with virtuous and honorable dispositions could find refuge there, for gatherings of such people fostered the creative interpersonal relationships that effect positive social transformation.

Because so many misshapen and malcontent citizens found their way into Renaissance monasteries and nunneries (according to Rabelais), only handsome nuns and monks could take part in the Abbey of Thélème, but they had to agree to remain the rest of their lives, or leave the community, after a one-year probationary period. Members were permitted to marry, acquire wealth, and live in liberty, as the name "Thélème" (freedom) infers. Well bred and highly educated, the Themelites possessed such noble dispositions that no moral law was needed to restrain them. There existed but a single commandment in the abbey: *"Do what thou wilt."*[9] Accordingly, Themelites ate, drank, worked, and slept only when inclined to do so, and they lived out lives of disciplined luxury in ample apartments with elegant appointments such as pleasure gardens and baths of myrrh. That simple elegance was reflected in their manner of dress, as well.[10] Although the abbey contained marvelous staircases and arcades, the real trophies were the beautiful libraries that preserved its Greek, Latin, Hebrew, French, Italian, and Spanish collections.

In the Abbey of Thélème, a model community where wealth was welcomed but not hoarded, not a single clock or sundial could be discovered on the premises to guide prayer schedules; mechanical time was altogether abolished.[11] Because the Themelites also lived free of all arbitrary laws, rules, and regulations—they honored individual volition and free will, remained in accord with nature, and strove toward virtue. As a refuge from error, only truth was spoken in the abbey. The Themelites broke the chains of oppression by recognizing the fact that we *"all engage in things forbidden, and yearn for things denied."*[12]

The convivial spirit of Pantagruelism that informs interpersonal relationships in the Abbey of Thélème reaches full expression in the third book. The hero Pantagruel, who lends his name to the philosophy of Pantagruelism, develops (in adulthood) a cheerful disposition that excuses deficiencies in others and a geniality that extends them welcome. Notwithstanding Frère Jean's martial spirit and Pantagruel's youthful transgressions, Pantagruelists strive to live nonviolently, in peace with their neighbors, and so sometimes they must flee from hypocrites, inquisitors, and calumniators,[13] an allusion to Rabelais's own escapes. Adherents of Pantagruelism are generally slow to anger or to find fault, and they attempt to interpret the folly of others in the best possible light. Pantagruelism is, in essence, a generous form of Christian charity that suffuses the third book.

Intriguingly, the philosophy of Pantagruelism has an analogue in the herb "pantagruelion," which grows upward of one and a half meters (five to six feet) in height, and the females produce seed-laden flowers. Rabelais depicts pantagruelion as a miraculous plant possessing more applications than are fully relatable. A natural fiber, pantagruelion was spun into hangmen's ropes, tablecloths, bed linens, and rigging for seagoing vessels. It also made an excellent fire-resistant asbestos and could be consumed as a mood-enhancing hashish; it also served as an important ingredient in the alchemical "philosopher's stone." When imbibed communally, the pantagruelion brought folks together in harmony and conferred upon them such powers that even the Olympian gods feared invasion of their celestial realms by devotees of the herb. [14]

Pantagruelion exhibits several "peculiar properties" that so complement its "many virtues, so many powers, such perfection, and so many wonderful effects," it might be elected by other plants the "wooden monarch to reign and dominate over them." Pantagruelion also possesses therapeutic medical properties, which include easing "tense sinews, contracted joints, podagric sclerosis and swellings caused by gout." Were that not sufficiently marvelous, pantagruelion could be applied to burns or be compounded into a "remedy for the gripe and convulsions in horses."[15] Following Pliny, Rabelais endowed the juice of the plant with the ability to kill ear parasites, and the pantagruelion suppresses semen in men "if eaten copiously and often." The pantagruelion is "sowed at the first return of the swallow; it is gathered in when the cicada begins to sound hoarse."[16]

The virtues of pantagruelion are so manifold and illustrious—so assorted and useful are its applications—that Pantagruel and the devilish Sophist Panurge pack plenty of pantagruelion for their long journey to consult the oracle of the Divine Bottle (*Dive Bouteille*) concerning Panurge's ill-advised wedding plans. They take along "both the green, untreated kind and the dressed and preserved" sort that kept longer.[17] The third book concludes with a cannabis song (in the style of Virgil's *Eclogues*) encouraging the spread of the heavenly pantagruelion herb:

> Indies, Sabia, Araby: take heed:
> Myrrh, incense, ebony, cease ye to praise,
> Accept our plant and bear away the seed,
> Sow it at home, a gift for all of your days
> If in your fields ye luckily it raise,
> Thanks to Heaven, thanks by the million,
> For France, wherein our happy plant doth breed;
> Blessed our realm for *pantagruelion*.[18]

Such a bucolic vision of social transformation finds a direct correlate in the utopian community of the Abbey of Thélème—for its doors, gates, windows, and gutters were fabricated from the hallowed pantagruelion plant. Although Rabelais never acknowledged that pantagruelion was hemp, that positive equivalence was made in the nineteenth century, when a keen public interest in Oriental hashish surfaced following the publication of Thomas De Quincey's autobiographical work *Confessions of an English Opium-Eater* in 1822. Although that book focuses on the effects of laudanum (opium and alcohol), the unexpected popularity of *Confessions* set the stage for extended exposés on the psychoactive effects of many other plants—including cannabis.

Members of the Hashish-Eaters Club (*Le Club des Hachichins*), a loose confederation of nineteenth-century artists and scientists, met monthly at the Pimodan Hotel in Paris. They wrote exuberant accounts of their experiments with mixtures of hashish, wine, and opium. The combined effects of those substances brought upon them hallucinations not normally associated with cannabis alone. Conceivably, their hashish preparations were strong enough to produce visions, but expectations concerning the effects of that exotic substance could have tainted their experiments (as might a placebo effect). In either case, some claims made by a few hashish-eaters concerning the extraordinary properties of cannabis as a strong psychedelic may seem exaggerated to readers in the contemporary world. Nonetheless, as we shall see, many of them point toward peak-experiences.

The French psychiatrist Jacques-Joseph Moreau first learned about the wonders of hashish while touring the Middle East during the 1830s. Becoming curious about its medical properties, he began treating his Arab patients with cannabis, and he observed very few adverse reactions in them. Having thus determined hashish to be an extremely safe substance (by the dubious ethical standards of the day), Dr. Moreau returned to Europe with enough hashish to continue investigating its pharmacological properties in hopes of finding better treatments for insomnia and depression. Personal reports concerning his own experimentations with hashish (taken in the form of a green paste similar to a full-extract cannabis oil) show his mind filled with phantasmagorical ideations, but he retained a conscious lucidity, a kind of hyper-awareness, that enabled him to reflect upon those experiences as they unfolded.

Before long Moreau was serving cannabis-laced confections (*dawa-mesk*) to some of his artist friends in France, including such notable personages as Alexander Dumas, Théophile Gautier, Victor Hugo, Honoré de Balzac, Gustave Flaubert, Gérard de Nerval, and Charles Baudelaire—many of whom were eager to explore the mental effects of hashish.[19] These gatherings, which sometimes included dinner, grew into the *Le Club des Hachichins*. Members met monthly in a paneled room rented by painter Fernand Boissard at the Pimodan Hotel, which featured a domed ceiling, yellowed glass windows, and a marbled mantelpiece. Adorning its walls were tapestries and paintings, and Egyptian statuettes were scattered about the room. The Orientalism of the décor (and sometimes the costumes), part of a fashion trend sweeping Western Europe at the time, aesthetically charged the meetings. Hashish perfectly suited the Orientalist sensibilities of the day, and Moreau delighted in offering cannabis paste confections to his guests from Oriental porcelain dishes in quasi-ritualistic ceremonies.

The hashish that Moreau later sourced from North Africa was frequently combined with finely ground almonds or pistachios, sugar, orange peel, spices, and sometimes opium. That preparation could be consumed as a paste eaten from a spoon, spread on bread or crackers, cooked into pastries, or served as part of a meal followed by strong black coffee (as was the custom in parts of the Orient). Still, not everyone who attended those *soirées* partook of Moreau's cannabis delectables; Gautier writes that Baudelaire's experimentations never led to a sustained engagement with hashish.[20] Those who did participate were asked to gauge, with considerable attention, how the cannabis effected their imaginations (since his callers were largely artists and intellectuals). As its effects wore off, discussions ensued that contrasted the properties of hashish with those of other psychoactive substances such as opium (more readily available than hashish and used widely as a medication).

Experimentations among members of the Hashish-Eaters Club were interdisciplinary collaborations that adhered to the methods of rational empirical investigation and drew from psychology, literature, and art. They had legitimate scientific, aesthetic, and philosophical dimensions.[21] Some members of the Hashish-Eaters Club generated sensational reports that spurred interest in cannabis—and the Orient more generally—among their readers.[22] The Hashish-Eaters did not always report the effects of hashish intoxication flatteringly. The essayist Théophile Gautier first chronicled the proceedings of the group initially in an addendum to Moreau's *Of Hashish and Mental Derangement*, but later more completely in "Le Club des Haschischins." In that extended treatment, Gautier describes Moreau as an enthusiastic hashish-eater who, as the dosages grew stronger, was the first to see "stars in his plate and the firmament at the bottom of the soup tureen; then he turned his face to the wall, speaking to himself and laughing loudly, his eyes shining, and in a jubilant mood."[23]

Gautier also reports several instances of mental clarity akin to what Abraham Maslow identified as peak-experiences. He notes synesthesia, for instance, a mix of sensory perceptions in which one "hears" colors and "sees" sounds:

> My sense of hearing had become abnormally acute. I could hear the very sounds of the colors. Sounds which were green, red, blue or yellow, reached my ears in perfectly distinct waves. An overturned glass, the creaking of an armchair, a whispered word, vibrated and echoed within me like peals of thunder. [. . .] Never had beatitude flooded me with its waves: I had so melted into the indefinable, I was so absent, so free from myself (that detestable witness ever dogging one's footsteps) that I realized for the first time what might be the way of life of elemental spirits, of angels, of souls separated from their bodies.[24]

Noting the fleeting nature of such epiphanies, Gautier concedes the hashish "takes you and leaves you" as it will, as if granting to one "lucid moments in a fit of madness."[25] On another such occasion, Gautier feels his body melt and become transparent, as if it were made of pure light. Elsewhere, he describes several fellow hash-eaters who roll on the ground in abandon and confused cries of: "God how happy I am! What bliss! I'm in ecstasy! In Paradise! I'm diving into abysses of delight!"[26] Some participants recounted seeing Elysian visions or having death and rebirth experiences (which have correlates in the Mystery cults and shamanistic practices explored in the preceding chapter).

Nineteenth-century experiments with hashish, such as those of the Hashish-Eaters, led many members of the reading public to erroneously conclude that hashish was stronger than opium. Such strained claims regarding the potency of cannabis may speak more to the scandalous nature of it in polite society at the time, overall misconceptions about its effects, or the ingestion of cannabis with other psychoactive agents (e.g., in a scented green paste made from Indian hemp, butter, and a small amount of opium). Misunderstandings and conflations, such as these, make it difficult to discern the psychoactive properties of hashish alone in the reports of Gautier, Baudelaire, and some of the other Hashish-Eaters. Baudelaire, for instance, became increasingly concerned about the negative consequences of sustained use of hashish, seemingly ignoring those of opium.[27]

For a short time, Baudelaire rented a room adjoining the one where the Hashish-Eaters held their revelries. The celebrated poet was young, popular, and rich, and his interludes with that band of psychedelic adventurers became the occasion for formal writings. Baudelaire penned an essay titled "On Wine and Hashish," and he innovated the genre of prose-poetry in "The Poem of Hashish," which he later integrated into his influential work *Artificial Paradises* (*Les paradis artificiels*). Baudelaire meanwhile busied himself with an impressionistic translation of De Quincey's *Confessions of an English Opium-Eater*.

In "On Wine and Hashish," a study contrasting those two substances (reminiscent of those undertaken by Arabic writers centuries earlier), Baudelaire confuses the effects of hashish and opium (which he took more often). He recognizes in these substances a similar rhapsodic quality, but he warns those seeking paradise through these plants that they risked creating their own hell (an ideological position that the writer Gustave Flaubert refuted).[28] Despite such admonitions, Baudelaire remained a stalwart devotee of Bacchus, and he became addicted to opium after it was prescribed to treat a stomach malady. In "The Poem of Hashish," Baudelaire portrays opium as a "peaceful charmer," while he denigrates hashish as a "far more fiendish" spirit. Yet, he observes contrariwise that cannabis sometimes "covers this mind with a magic lustre, colors it in solemnity and lights all of its depths," so that "everything, the very universality of existence rises up before you in unimagined glory."[29]

In other accounts of hashish intoxication, Baudelaire notes how cannabis improves his mental acuity significantly: it "sharpens the senses and the powers of perception, of taste, sight, smell, hearing—all participate equally in this progression. The eyes pierce the infinite. The ear hears sounds that are almost imperceptible amid even the most tumultuous din."[30] Baudelaire identifies lucid intervals lasting only a minute or more in an otherwise interminable fantasy, which he characterizes as a kind of self-forgetting. While he would not understand them as such, the following passage from "The Poem of Hashish" recounts a peak-experience in which he sees directly into the luminous nature of things. Baudelaire writes:

> You stare at a tree that harmoniously rocks in the breeze; in a few seconds what would for the poet be a natural comparison becomes a reality to you. You endow the tree with your passions and desires; its capriciously swaying limbs become your own, so that soon you yourself *are* that tree. Thus, when looking skyward, you behold a bird soaring into the deep azure. At first, the bird seems to *represent* the immortal yearning to soar above earthly concerns. But you have already become that bird. Imagine that you are seated, smoking a pipe. Your attention lingers a moment too long on the spirals of bluish clouds that drift upward from the pipe's bowl.[31]

Under the influence of hashish (and other intoxicants), Baudelaire notes that the most trivial things take on an extraordinary intensity. He cites, for support, the remarks of one "nervous August Bedloe" who swallowed a great quantity of opium before setting off on his morning walk. That normally unremarkable event suddenly became a scintillating experience in which a whole universe of suggestion came in "the quivering of a leaf—in the hue of a blade of grass—in the shape of a trefoil—in the humming of a bee—in the gleaming of a dewdrop—in the breathing of the wind—in the faint odors that came from the forest."[32] The beauty of nature stirs the mystical soul toward epiphanic experiences that are exceedingly meaningful. For this reason, Baudelaire employs quasireligious language to describe his own peak-experiences, though holding fast to a clinical detachment and the rigorous method of observation.

The young Fitz Hugh Ludlow, like Charles Baudelaire, drew inspiration from De Quincey's *Confessions of an English Opium-Eater*. A member of the Union College graduating class of 1856, Ludlow found unexpected fame at twenty-one years of age for his own interrogation of consciousness, which he published (with little revision) under the sensational and quirky title *The Hasheesh Eater: Being Passages from the Life of a Pythagorean*. A cautionary tale written by a religiously minded young man inspired by the Christian revivalism then sweeping the United States, *The Hasheesh Eater* is an autobiographical narrative. In it, Ludlow chronicles his journey toward Christian salvation alongside multiple attempts to reform his cannabis tincture habit of three to four years in duration.

Without question, Fitz Hugh Ludlow was an American original: a precocious adolescent hashish-eater who experimented with cannabis in isolation at a time when there was no cultural context for such psychological expeditions. One scholar calls him a small-scale Timothy Leary who turned Union College students on to cannabis,[33] yet Ludlow also chronicled college life during the 1850s when a wave of secularization gave birth to the public higher education movement. In fact, he was admired and liked among his fellow classmates, and by tipping some of them to the virtues of hashish, he discovered that its effects varied depending on personality type and social surroundings. Extreme personalities felt it most acutely, while more passive types generally noticed little or no influence from the hashish.[34] He wrote about those experimentations at a time when marijuana was still unfamiliar to most Americans.

Ludlow first encountered cannabis at the establishment of a Poughkeepsie apothecary in the form of an olive-brown paste the consistency of pitch. A curious lad of seventeen studying theology in upstate New York, he consulted James F. Johnston's *Chemistry of Common Life* and found therein a historical overview of cannabis and its therapeutic applications, as well as a description of the narcotic value of its resinous flowers. At that time, no drugs were illegal in the United States, and chloroform and later cocaine were freely available. As an herbal remedy, cannabis entered the American pharmacopoeia during the 1850s (as Ludlow was writing); soon thereafter, all manner of hemp medicines became legally purchasable in pharmacies across the United States—although the popularity of medical cannabis waned in the early twentieth century with the advent of synthetic medications.

Moreau may have first recognized the efficacy of cannabis in alleviating headaches, stimulating appetite, and bringing on sleep, but William Brooke O'Shaughnessy discovered the anticonvulsive properties of the plant when he conducted research as a physician in India. Tinctures of cannabis made their debut in London a decade before they were sold lawfully in the United States (under the name "Tilden's Extract"). Deemed effective in treating alcoholism, opiate addiction, anthrax, rabies, and tetanus, cannabis tinctures varied greatly in strength from batch to batch, and if not well shaken, the last dropper reportedly could cause intense psychedelic experiences in unsuspecting users. As a matter of course, all manner of marijuana preparations were sold without prescription in Europe and the United States from the mid-nineteenth century into the first decades of the twentieth century; nearly thirty pharmaceutical cannabis preparations were available in the American marketplace when their sale became practically impossible (following the Marihuana Tax Act of 1937).[35]

On account of his sickly constitution, Ludlow kept abreast of the latest medical innovations by reading widely. Not put off by warnings concerning the dangers of cannabis advanced by his apothecaries, he repeatedly experimented with marijuana before being sent to Princeton by his father (a converted Calvinist who worked in the emancipation movement). Finding himself a member of the junior class at Union College in 1855, on account of demission from Princeton due to fire, Ludlow lived on campus in a small town of just eight thousand souls. He quickly located a chemist who sold "Tilden's Extract" and solid preparations of cannabis.[36] Under their influence, Ludlow recorded demonic visions of shadows and corpses reminiscent of the imagery that he so admired in the stories of Edgar Allan Poe.

An excursion to Niagara Falls following his graduation provided the backdrop for a series of profound peak-experiences recounted in *The Hasheesh Eater*. He describes feelings of awe before the majesty of the falls, and he attempts to convey to his readers the true moments of unutterable calm and inner communication with heaven that he experienced there. The spiritual openings stimulated by the falls were cannabis fueled, and they enthused him to write a poem of celebration in which he marvels at the power of the rapids, and the colossal descent of the rushing waters into the quiet river below. Rather than try to raise his own puny voice above the mighty roar of Niagara Falls, Ludlow decides to "keep silence where God speaks" rather than dim His glory with words. The mystical sublimity of the scene leaves a "permanency of impressions" on the mind of the young writer—ones that faded with time, but were never completely lost.[37] In a nod to the ineffable, Ludlow notes the unutterability of the rapture that he felt at Niagara and asserts that it defies the human capacity for communication.

Following the success of *The Hasheesh Eater*, Ludlow became a poet, cultural critic, journalist, novelist, and travel writer. Tragically, ill health and financial difficulties hounded him until his death at age thirty-four from tuberculosis—a disease for which he was first prescribed opium.

Though Ludlow battled with dependence on stronger substances (including morphine) late in his brief life, his writings on cannabis reinforced the nineteenth-century notion of hashish as a powerful psychedelic. Yet, Ludlow refused to reject cannabis wholesale, and he included editorial essays on the therapeutic value of hashish (surprisingly in agreement with contemporary American views about marijuana medicine). In the end, Ludlow concluded that cannabis also facilitates transcendental experiences akin to those outlined in Ralph Waldo Emerson's essay *Nature*. Under its influence, Ludlow observes, one may discover in the natural world "the most startling illustrations and incarnations of spiritual facts."[38]

Louise May Alcott, another nineteenth-century American writer with an interest in cannabis, served as a nurse during the Civil War. Her duties caring for hundreds of men in various states of suffering, disease, and dying at the Union Hotel Hospital in Georgetown were so strenuous that she was stricken with what was diagnosed as a form of pneumonia (but which may have been typhoid fever). When Alcott returned home with a prescription for laudanum to treat her illness, she was already familiar with the curative effects of cannabis and its ability to lighten mood, for it sold locally for just six cents a stick.[39] The enthusiastic reception of her novel *Little Women* turned Alcott into a celebrity author of juvenile fiction overnight, but unbeknownst to most of her readers, she maintained a secret literary life composing sensational narratives, including some in which cannabis played a central part.

Alcott published her melodramatic works anonymously or under the pseudonym A. M. Barnard, and she earned from them between twenty-five to a hundred dollars apiece. Writing these short stories provided her with an alternate venue for perfecting her craft, and she seems to have particularly enjoyed penning those that drew from personal experience. Playfully, *Little Women* contains autobiographical clues through which the sharp-witted reader might discover the hidden allusions that she carefully embedded to authenticate the true authorship of her commercial work. The decipherment of those clues led to the recovery of a considerable body of material by the writer.[40] The fact that "Perilous Play" and other works were not attributable to her pen until the 1940s speaks to her success in subtly hinting at authorship (as they remained unattributable for decades).

In her short story "The Perilous Play," Alcott puts cannabis at the heart of the plot. Since any association with its true author threatened to cut short her bourgeoning career as a writer of adolescent fiction, it was published anonymously in 1869. The story features a cast of indolent socialites chock full of the ennui that sometimes typifies those born into the moneyed class. On one such day of unrelenting boredom, Belle Daventry cries out for any "new and interesting amusement" (as days and nights filled with gossip, card playing, and croquet have lost their allure). At that very moment, the Spanish beauty and heroine of the story, Rose St. Just, happens to be reading the legend of the Lotus Eaters (devotees of a narcotic that induces peaceful lethargy). The title gives the young and handsome Dr. Meredith a smashing idea. He pulls out an exquisite little box made of tortoise shell and gold and proposes provocatively to the jaded Belle: "Eat six of these despised bonbons, and you *will* be amused in a new, delicious, and wonderful manner."[41] When she inquires what makes them so special, the good doctor replies that they are hashish confections. He normally consumes twenty or more, and so he offers Belle ten bonbons—a delicate bit of diplomacy that she finds convincing.

Spying the sultry Miss St. Just alone, Dr. Meredith offers her a "taste of Elysium" and places six bonbons on her book. He convincingly adds that he uses hashish on his patients as a remedy for nervous disorders, a common affliction among aristocratic ladies. Initially she declines, but when her friends query the doctor regarding the effects of the hashish that they have just eaten, he assures the group that they will be "in a seraphic state of mind" within a few hours.[42] A short time later, Belle is laughing frequently and pleasantly, while Norton becomes incredibly loquacious— another welcome change. Any story needs a good plot twist, and it is discovered with dismay that Belle Daventry went sailing while under the influence of hashish. Suspecting that their friend sought refuge from an unexpected storm at a nearby lighthouse, the dashing Mr. Done, emboldened by his own consumption of hashish bonbons, rushes out onto the water to search for the missing lady (accompanied by Rose).

Once adrift, Mr. Done dramatically confesses a long-concealed love for the shocked Rose. He begs her to profess her feelings for him in return: "I am mad, Rose," he shouts, "with love—and hashish!"[43] They enter the tempest, but Mr. Done grows increasingly distrustful of his ability to operate the boat when the effects of the laced bonbons reach their height. Rose helps him fight off a dreadful drowsiness, which leaves him feeling lost, as if he were in a dream. When he begs softly for a kiss, Rose admits that she, too, furtively ate of the hashish confections and admits to a secret love for Mr. Done. Thus roused from his stupor, he clutches the oars and, with her at the helm, they make for the lighthouse with renewed vigor. Dripping, but elated to be dragged to safety by the keeper, the couple remain at the lighthouse until the storm passes. Somewhat timid about having spent the night together when they return the next morning, in the end, the "dangerous experiment" with hashish not only rescues everyone from boredom, but Mr. Done gains the courage to confess his love—and Rose the temerity to return it. "Heaven bless hashish," Mr. Done declares, "if its dreams end like this!"[44]

Possibly due to the fact that Louise May Alcott was an abolitionist, feminist, and the daughter of transcendentalists, many of her sensational stories emphasize strong female characters and explored alternate states of consciousness, including those brought about by opium and hashish. In addition to being professionally satisfying, she found such writing an important emotional outlet, notwithstanding her legitimate fears of attribution.[45] The full body of her work, now available to scholars and laypersons, establishes her reputation as an artist adept at depicting complex human emotion within the genre limitations of the sensational and sentimental, the realistic and the gothic, and the domestic drama and psychological thriller.

At the turn of the twentieth century, a new generation of writers was coming of age and they extended the literary explorations of Gautier, Baudelaire, Ludlow, Alcott, and others. Among these authors were Aleister Crowley, William Butler Yeats, and Walter Benjamin, each of whom responded uniquely to the forces of mechanization unleashed in the wake of the Industrial Revolution. They attested to profound shifts in human relations in which urban dwellers keenly felt psychological isolation and fragmentation resulting from severed social and familial bonds. The lower and middle classes endured exploitation by corporate barons and capitalist magnates of the Gilded Age. In response to alarmingly wide disparities between the rich and working poor, labor unions formed to shield workers from the grossest abuses (such as child labor).

Into this transitional and turbulent period, Aleister Crowley was born. By all accounts an odd little boy, he grew into a highly eccentric fellow whose decadent lifestyle left his British well-to-do evangelical (Plymouth Brethren) family flabbergasted. Baptized Edward Alexander, young Alick was always sickly. His relatives feared that the boy would not live to see adulthood on account of kidney disease. His poor health probably contributed to a morbid interest in death, obsession with the occult, and general perversity of character. From a young age Aleister (as he would later rename himself) was brooding, highly intelligent, and an avid reader. He became infatuated as an adolescent with acts of transgression (sin), rebellion, and the possibility of redemption from them—areas of inquiry that later led him to train as a ceremonial magician in an esoteric tradition whose notable members included Paracelsus, Agrippa, and Cagliostro.[46]

When he turned eighteen, Crowley inherited fifty thousand pounds from his father's estate (which he squandered in due course) and left home to study literature and philosophy at Cambridge University. Once there, he began to publish his poetry, but another brief bout of illness inspired him to undertake neophyte induction into the secret Hermetic Order of the Golden Dawn after his recovery. Yoga, sexual intercourse, ritual magic, drugs, and alchemy soon became regular facets of his exploration of consciousness. Evidently adept at such pursuits, he was swiftly promoted to the rank of *Zelator*, *Practicus*, and *Philosophus* in fairly rapid succession. However, his libertine lifestyle and bisexuality irked some members of the Golden Dawn, including the celebrated poet William Butler Yeats—an initiate also anxious to climb ranks in the secret group. Ignoring all howls of indignation, Crowley went on to develop a religious philosophy known as Thelema in his *Liber AL vel Legis* (*The Book of the Law*), which made "*Do what thou wilt*" its main creed (a bow to Rabelais's abbey, of course).

Crowley openly repudiated his family's Christian values along with the stolid status quo, and he instead pursued a unified perception beyond the dualities of good and evil—a state of awareness known in the Golden Dawn as "Genius" (in other traditions the Higher Self, the Silent Watcher, Adonai, Logos, Vishnu, Buddhahood, the Great One).[47] Although he strayed far outside of the moral compass of the British bourgeoisie, some of his occult practices have correlates in the shamanistic traditions and Mystery religions that we encountered earlier. Crowley even publicly offered the Rites of Eleusis at Caxton Hall in Westminster, and his recreation of them focused on raising the spiritual consciousness of the audience so as "to induce religious ecstasy in the highest form" among the masses.[48]

Like Baudelaire, and Ludlow before him, Crowley poured through De Quincey's *Confessions of an English Opium-Eater*, and it inspired him to study the medical applications of opium, hashish, and cocaine alongside a new Bayer Company product called heroin (widely reputed to be more effective than morphine for pain management). Crowley also wrote about his experiments with cannabis in the essays "The Psychology of Hashish" and "The Most Holy Grass of the Arabs." In order to learn more about other spiritual traditions, he undertook a series of international excursions that led him to Egypt to study Sufism and gain some fluency in Arabic, Burma to learn meditation techniques, Mexico to acquire shamanic powers, and India to investigate Shaivism and train in yoga. Yeats not only competed with him as a member of the Golden Dawn, but also shared some of Crowley's interests in mythology and the occult.

The fondness Yeats developed for myth and fairytale led him to the work of the poet-painter William Blake, whom he helped to recover as an important Romantic poet and visual artist who anticipated the Modernism of the twentieth century. From Blakean theories regarding the fragmentary nature of the unenlightened mind (outlined in his poems "Four Zoas" and "Jerusalem"), Yeats discovered the writings of the philosopher Emanuel Swedenborg and Christian mystic Jakob Böhme, two main influences on the highly idiosyncratic mythologies that Blake developed in his prophetic works. Yeats next moved on to the Society for Psychic Research, where he met Madame Blavatsky, the controversial cofounder of the Theosophical Society dedicated to understanding esoteric religious teachings such as the Cabala. (That society chose the young Jiddu Krishnamurti as the World Teacher, and although he publicly relinquished that role in 1929, Krishnamurti continued to teach and write until his death.)

Yeats's persistent interest in magic and alchemy drew him into the Hermetic Order of the Golden Dawn through its appropriation of Rosicrucian and cabbalistic symbolism (such as the rose and Tree of Life). By his own admission, Yeats felt that his poetry benefited from every phase of his religious studies and occult activities—and that taking hashish along with several "followers of the eighteenth century mystic Saint-Martin" contributed to his ultimate understanding that revelation comes from the self.[49] During that session, Yeats observed some of the mystic's followers smoking and dancing, while others talked wildly, until three women came to retrieve their (apparently) wayward male relatives.

In his final years, Yeats fully embraced Eastern philosophy after spiritual experiences such as that above (which hashish assisted in opening). Perhaps a testament to his attainment, the great poet collaborated on a translation of the *Upanishads* with Shree Purohit. In their rendition of that seminal Hindu text (belonging to the Vedānta), we sense that Yeats's religious journey culminated in the unitive consciousness that comes with peak experiences. Yeats and Purohit translate opening lines from the *Easha-Upanishad*:

That is perfect. This is perfect. Perfect comes from perfect. Take perfect from perfect, the remainder is perfect.
May peace and peace and peace be everywhere.
Whatever lives is full of the Lord. Claim nothing; enjoy, do not covet His property.
Then hope for a hundred years of life doing your duty. No other way can prevent deeds from clinging, proud as you are of your human life.
They that deny the Self, return after death to a godless birth, blind, enveloped in darkness.
The Self is one. Unmoving, it moves faster than the mind. The senses lag, but Self runs ahead. Unmoving it outruns pursuit. Out of Self comes the breath that is the life of all things.
Unmoving, it moves; is far away, yet near; within all, outside all.
Of a certainty the man who can see all creatures in himself, himself in all creatures, knows no sorrow.
How can a wise man, knowing the unity of life, seeing all creatures in himself, be deluded or sorrowful?
The Self is everywhere, without a body, without a shape, whole, pure, wise, all-knowing, far shining, self-depending, all transcending; in the eternal procession assigning to every period its proper duty. [50]

In light of Yeats's lengthy explorations in mythology, magic, religion, and mysticism, how interesting to see him working this rich material for his own spiritual benefit, as well as that of other Westerners (who might encounter this Hindu scripture only as a consequence of the translators' fame).

By the 1920s and 1930s in the West, social attitudes about cannabis, coca, opium, mescaline, and other such substances became much more conservative, resulting in changes to criminal law and government policy that subjected those plants to strict regulation. The overall effect of that clampdown on hitherto legal medicines was to dissuade all but the most determined individuals from exploring religious experience through them. The cultural theorist Walter Benjamin bucked that trend and sought out mind-altering substances for personal experimentation after reading about them. His studies of cannabis struck a more scientific and empirical note than those by members of *Le Club des Hachichins*, Crowley, or

Yeats, for Benjamin kept careful records (or "protocols") of therapeutic sessions that took place between 1927 and 1934 in Berlin, Marseilles, and Ibiza. As part of his study of consciousness-raising substances, he ate hashish, smoked opium, and allowed himself to be injected with mescaline and the sedative eucodal simultaneously.[51] Some of his protocols were recorded while under the influence—others written down after the effects of such "cocktails" wore off. When others participated in them, such as the philosopher Ernst Bloch, their voices spoke directly to the reader.

Although Benjamin planned to write a book on hashish, which he thought would be revolutionary, that project never reached completion; it comes down to us only in fragments. In his scattered records and notes, Benjamin (who developed a keen interest in Jewish mysticism) argues that cannabis opened for him new pathways to aesthetic, philosophical, and political insights. Metaphysically speaking, he shared with Aldous Huxley a fascination with the nondual reconfiguration of the subject-object binary (which defines so much of ordinary consciousness),[52] and so Benjamin used the German word *Rausch* to designate an all-consuming state of intoxication whose outcome was the highest intellectual clarity that one could attain. Although generally rendered into English as "intoxication" (or "trance"), the noun *Rausch* derives from an onomatopoeic verb meaning "to rustle; rush; roar; thunder."[53] Inspired by Baudelaire's *Artificial Paradises* to consume hashish, Benjamin altered the term *Rausch* to make it denote the thrilling state of consciousness encountered during every cannabis protocol and in experiments with other consciousness-altering substances. Many of those protocols provide accounts of transcendental peak-experiences.

On one such occasion in September 1928, Benjamin was inspired to take hashish after reading Hermann Hesse's *Steppenwolf*. In Marseilles at the time, Benjamin walked outside into the evening and stubbornly fixed his gaze on the faces that he encountered, "some of which were of remarkable coarseness or ugliness." Suddenly, it dawned on Benjamin that for the true artist such hideousness hides a reservoir of true beauty (behind deep wrinkles and worried brows). Rather than continuing to denounce outward appearances, Benjamin starts to recognize a kinship in each passing face—an intuitive perception that left no question of his ever feeling lonely again. He recalls a "deeply submerged feeling of happiness" coming upon him that elevated enraptured prosaic beings "to the highest power."[54] Under the influence of hashish, he discovered a state of being whereby he became free of all desire—and therefore incapable of fear.

That Benjamin came to such significant spiritual realizations during his lifetime is a great benediction in light of his tragic and premature death. A Jewish man fleeing from the Nazis on foot through the Pyrenees in 1940, Benjamin died by his own hand (it appears via a morphine overdose) near the French and Spanish border, rather than suffer internment and possible transfer to a concentration camp. However, mystery still surrounds Benjamin's death, as he was in possession of an entry visa to the United States—and the next day the border crossing reopened.[55] World War II ended five years later, and a new generation of writers and intellectuals came forth to push the boundaries of public consciousness. As quickening technological innovation linked disparate parts of the world and sped transportation among them during the 1950s and 1960s, authors and critics heralded a new impulse toward democratization and global citizenship—and their challenge to the conservative mores of their day inspired countercultural revolutions whose aftershocks would be felt in societies around the globe.

Allen Ginsberg was among the foremost of those intellectuals challenging postwar values in the United States. Alongside a cadre of authors closely associated with the Beat Generation (including Jack Kerouac, William Burroughs, Gary Snyder, Lawrence Ferlinghetti, and Gregory Corso), Ginsberg turned nonconformity into an art. Together, these artists helped to liberalize social values, generate interest in religious studies (particularly Hindu and Buddhist), and to redefine sexuality; they also made a case for rejecting Western materialism and consumerism, scrutinizing the exploitative nature of global capitalism, and rethinking bans on consciousness-raising plants (including cannabis) and synthetic substances (such as LSD). The Beats provided inspiration for the agitations of counterculture revolutionaries (championing women's liberation, civil rights, free speech, and world peace) during the 1960s and 1970s, before a return to social conservatism followed the election of President Ronald Reagan in 1980.

A Blakean like Yeats, Ginsberg's poem "Howl" landed like a bombshell in the oppressively conformist America of the mid-1950s. It was as radical for its day as *The Marriage of Heaven and Hell* in the eighteenth century. The poem's long riffs reminiscent of jazz gave flight to lyrical yet stinging denunciations of postwar urban existence, which for a large underclass meant poverty, desperation, addiction, vanished prospects, and simmering rage against the oppressor and his institutions. Like James Joyce's *Ulysses* decades earlier, "Howl" was banned as pornographic before being exonerated at trial as a work of art and social critique. The media frenzy surrounding those court proceedings turned the unkempt bohemian with sparkling eyes and a ready chant into one of the most provocative figures of the day—and the full body of his work would make significant contributions to American literature and culture.

In the 1965 essay "First Manifesto to End the Bringdown," Ginsberg writes to the general public concerning "the actual experience of the smoked herb," for he felt that there existed too many misconceptions in the country regarding the actual psychoactive properties of cannabis. Perusing it fifty years later, one is struck by Ginsberg's clear apprehension of the religious and medical attributes of marijuana, his alarm about environmental degradation, and his thoughts regarding the ongoing evolution of human beings. Writing from "San Francisco, California, USA, Kosmos," Ginsberg opens his manifesto by astutely noting: "marijuana consciousness is one that, ever so gently, shifts the center of attention *from* habitual shallow purely verbal guidelines and repetitive secondhand ideological interpretations of experience to more direct, slower, absorbing, occasionally microscopically minute, engagement with sensing phenomena during the high moments or hours after one has smoked." He suggests that although a minority of those who partake find the effect displeasing and make propaganda against the plant, most people around the world who have inhaled several breaths of it quickly adjust to the sensation of time slowing down. With a smidgeon of natural curiosity, Ginsberg counsels, cannabis opens an important and "useful area of mind-consciousness to be familiar with." Smoking marijuana, he contends, "is no more disrupting than Insight."[56]

A world traveler with a keen interest in spirituality and culture, he recalls smoking ganja in a circle of devotees, yogis, and Shaivite worshippers at Nimtalah Ghat in Calcutta and singing praise songs all night. In that religious context, cannabis was "considered a beginning of saddhana" (or yogic discipline). Ginsberg observes that all of India, Africa, and the Arab world "is familiar with ganja," at least as much as "high-minded but respectable 19th-century circles" were in Paris and London (e.g., *Le Club des Hachichins*). To reinforce that critical point, Ginsberg recounts sitting in Morocco under the generous shade of trees sipping mint tea and passing the kif pipe with old gentlemen and peaceable youths. He juxtaposes that cannabis experience with the suppression of black marijuana culture in the United States—noting the important relationship of blues, jazz, and other forms of black music to a history of religious cannabis use among African tribes and nations. Accordingly, Ginsberg denounces the prohibition of marijuana in the United States as a major and unconscious method for the repression of black rights. [57]

A poet, performance artist, and cultural critic, Ginsberg found cannabis useful in stimulating "specific optical and aural aesthetic perceptions," and he felt that it helped to sustain extended periods of concentrated activity, such as writing. He once professed to intuitively apprehend the inner structure of jazz music and classical composition under its influence—an epiphany that remained imprinted on his everyday consciousness. Ginsberg discovers the same perceptual effects at work in his appreciation of art; Cezanne's use of three-dimensional space seemed more evident and compelling. He recalls peak-experiences during some cannabis sessions and felt overcome by a tremendous awe that remained a permanent feature of his aesthetic sensibility. Owing to these and other artistic insights while taking cannabis, Ginsberg defiantly—and surprisingly—asserts that "most of the major (best and most famous too)" poets, painters, musicians, sculptors, actors, singers, and publishers "in America and England have been smoking marihuana for years and years." [58] Such a declaration frees him to rail again against the criminalization of cannabis, which he thought filled American jails with nonviolent offenders, often minorities, and supported an illegal black market for the plant's sale and distribution.

The broadminded nature of Ginsberg's plea for legalization is evident in his supposition that "future generations will have to rely on new faculties of awareness, rather than on new versions of old idea-systems" to cope with the complexities of globalization. He posits that a "new consciousness, or a new awareness will evolve to meet a changed ecological environment" and that the youth movements of the mid-1960s bear testament to its commencement. He cites an unprecedented familiarity with East Asian Buddhism, Indian yoga, and indigenous American shamanism among young people of that decade, and he evidences their new music of "hitherto unheard-of frankness and beauty" as proof of that evolution. [59] In the "First Manifesto to End the Bringdown," Ginsberg commends cannabis as an agent of self-awareness, self-transformation, and imagination vital to humanity and the arts, and he argued that continued prohibition of the plant is a moral, religious, and cultural outrage.

If Ginsberg positively glosses the social, intellectual, and spiritual revolutions taking place across the United States during the 1960s, then Joan Didion elucidates their shortcomings and warns of their excesses. She borrows the title of her influential collection of essays *Slouching toward Bethlehem* from Yeats's "The Second Coming." That choice makes California in the mid-to-late-1960s into an illustration of anarchy let loose upon the world—a place where the center no longer holds. While admitting to some positive social contributions by the hippie generation that followed the Beats, such as counter values esteeming nature and fostering an interest in being rather than becoming, Didion accuses them of too often devolving into carnivalesque hedonism. Her book of essays offers up a series of impressionistic vignettes upon which she bases that trenchant critique of California youth culture.

The title essay in *Slouching toward Bethlehem* skeptically appraises the Haight-Ashbury district of San Francisco where the hippie movement first took shape. She describes a place "where the social hemorrhaging was showing up" in the form of "missing children" gathering and calling themselves "hippies." She searches for characters like Deadeye, whom she discovers asleep at three in the afternoon with someone else crashed on his couch, and a girl "asleep on the floor beneath a poster of Allen Ginsberg."[60] The room is overheated; the young woman is sick. The scene shifts, and somewhere else in the Bay Area Max and Don share a joint in the car on the way to North Beach. In another place and time, Steve opines, he found love on LSD then lost it—only to recover it again with "nothing but grass." Elsewhere still, Otto is greatly relieved to discover that it was not the cocaine-and-wheat that made him ill, but "the chicken pox he caught baby-sitting for Big Brother and the Holding Company,"[61] a local band featuring the vocal heroics of Janis Joplin.

Didion's depictions of the hippie scene are unflinching, if sometimes skewed. When Max, Tom, and Sharon take LSD together in the living room, Barbara decides to smoke hashish alone in her bedroom as the other three trip out. Four hours pass without a sound when Max abruptly and cryptically proclaims: "Wow." Some days later, Sharon and Max hook up, and Barbara gets on "the woman's trip" (meaning that she keeps house, bakes, and works a few hours a week). Didion encounters this phrase repeatedly in her travels, and she ponders the paradoxical mingling of "nothin'-says-lovin'-like-something-from-the-oven" with the *Feminine Mystique*. How is it possible, Didion wonders, "for people to be the unconscious instruments of values they would strenuously reject on a conscious level," but she does not voice her thoughts to Barbara.[62] The final image in *Slouching toward Bethlehem* is one of the most enduring and critical of hippie dissipations: a five-year-old child flopped on a living room floor wearing white lipstick and "a reefer coat, reading a comic book"—on acid.[63] Oh, man.

In contrast to Ginsberg and Didion, Paul Bowles and Terry Southern put forth alternate visions of the role of cannabis in mid-to-late-twentieth-century American culture; one pens a marijuana morality tale and the other a parable of racial reconciliation (albeit one tinged with the racism of the era). Bowles's Oriental fairytale takes up the literary rivalry between cannabis and hemp that we saw play out in Islamic poetry and in essays by members of the Hashish-Eaters Club. In "The Story of Lahcen and Idir," the character of Lahcen stands for drink while Idir represents kif—their respective intoxicants of choice. The relative moral merit of each substance forms the basis of the parable. The title of the collection, *100 Camels in the Courtyard*, tacitly acknowledges the advantages of cannabis by alluding to the Arabic proverb: "A pipeful of kif before breakfast gives a man the strength of a hundred camels in the courtyard."

Although the subplots of this cannabis fable are interwoven, the narrative begins with two friends, Lahcen and Idir, who spot a beautiful girl on the beach in Merkala, Tangier. Her *djellaba* (loose outer robe) blows in the wind, and she wears no veil. Although young, all of her teeth are made of gold. Idir (kif) listens as Lahcen (alcohol) plans to take her for a walk and make a reality of his lecherous thoughts. The next morning, red-eyed and hung over, Lahcen explains that he decided not to accost the girl after all, but got smashed instead. Still a bit tipsy, and therefore uncharacteristically generous, Lahcen gives a gold ring to Idir worth fifty dirhams (over his friend's loud protests). The present was significant, as there was no work for young people, and the two scraped by.

Unfortunately for Idir, wine is cheap in Merkala, but his kif is costly. As a result, he learns to stay home and smoke by himself in the evenings. On one such occasion, Idir sees a small white-headed bird with black and white wings enter his room through an open window, and it prances about on the floor. There the creature remains for hours, seemingly contentedly.

When Idir strokes its head with his thumb, he impulsively slips Lahcen's ring around the neck of the bird, and of course it flies away with the treasure. Drunk when he hears the news, Lahcen becomes angry, and so Idir gives him a pair of used leather shoes (which after several misfortunes Lahcen sells for just ten dirhams). The animosity that develops between the friends comes to a head when the boys make a play on the same Muslim girl; they fight it out, but because Lahcen "was always drunk,"[64] Idir easily wins the day along with the lass (who seems perfectly pleased to go with the hashish smoker instead of the boozer).

Contrarily, the story "Red Dirt Marihuana" by Terry Southern sounds a sentimental note regarding cannabis culture in the South, but it highlights the continuing racism that has sullied the American experiment in democracy since the country's founding. In that narrative, a twelve-year-old white child named Harold brings a pillowcase full of marijuana to C. K., a black man twenty years his senior and the keeper of considerable wisdom regarding that herb's consciousness-raising properties. When Harold places the contents of the pillowcase on an old sheet of newspaper in front of him, C. K. queries the boy: "What you doin', Hal', bringin' in the *crop*?" C. K. inspects the dried buds, breaks them open, and tries to teach Harold to appreciate their fresh clean fragrance. They discover the cannabis together.

Quietly fishing one afternoon, they observe a cow alone, lying on its stomach, in a section of pastureland where the other members of the herd rarely venture. Its head is outstretched, and it contentedly chews cud. Impatient at the sight of such a docile creature, Harold remarks: "I ain't never seen no loco-weed make a cow act like *that*." C. K., however, understands that the happy creature stumbled upon some superior grass, and he explains to the boy that wild cannabis plants thriving in red clay dirt is most unusual. Excited at the prospect of a new project, Harold wants to dry and sell the marijuana; rather than take the risk, they sensibly decide to air the herbs among the branches of some sycamore trees. From that harvest, C. K. takes out two cigarette papers and rolls up a smoke, which he consumes with relish in front of the curious preteen. He next sorts the leaves, stems, flowers, and seeds—all the while explaining the benefits of doing so to the youngster.

An anxious Harold plies C. K. with questions about the effects of cannabis, which C. K. attempts to answer (implying that the earthy values of black rural life in Texas trump those of the white middle class). Seated cross-legged in a sagacious meditative posture with his back straight, C. K. concludes succinctly: "Boy, I done *tole* you," he whispers, "it feels *good*." If that's the case, Harold wonders aloud, why is it illegal, "if it's so all-fired good?" C. K. admits that he has pondered that insightful question himself, and he believes that it is not because marijuana makes white boys like Hal' sick. Uncertain if the youngster is old enough to understand, C. K. offers his own rationale for the prohibition of marijuana in the United States: "it's cause a man *see* too much when he git high, that's what. He see right *through* ever'thing." C. K. elaborates on that point, observing: "they's a lotta' trickin' an' lyin' go on in the world . . . they's a lotta ole *bull-crap* go on in the world" and when someone gets high, he or she "see right through there into the *truth* of it!" C. K. concludes that cannabis is illegal, not because it is harmful, but because those who imbibe it experience expanded perceptions that are not always welcomed by society. It makes people more independently minded. Noting that "ain't nothin' like good gage give a man the strength of patience," C. K. asks Hal', "you wan me to twist up a couple for *you*?" Reflecting for a moment, Hal' agrees reluctantly, adding with a bigotry indicative of the white south, "you let *me* lick'em though, dang it, C. K."[65]

Other contemporary literary explorations of cannabis and peak-experiences include *Great Jones Street*, the third novel by chronicler of all things Americana, Don DeLillo. When the marijuana-toking protagonist Bucky Wunderlick quits a successful rock tour midway, disenchanted with performing in front of hypnotized crowds of adoring fans, he unexpectedly becomes more famous. Because he cannot return to his mountain studio without the bothersome paparazzi of his rabid fan club interfering, Bucky retreats to a rundown flat on Great Jones Street in Manhattan where his girlfriend Opel lives. Unbeknown to Wunderlick, Opel arranges for the Mountain Tapes—secret recordings that capture a lost authenticity in his vocals and lyrics—to arrive at her place as a birthday surprise for the retiring singer. Before he can receive them, though, Opel dies of ill health.

When a bizarre group of the maverick artist's admirers, known collectively as Happy Valley Farm Commune, send a girl named Skippy as an emissary bearing a plain brown package containing a new wonder drug, it complicates Bucky's life considerably. As other fringe organizations catch wind of the mysterious substance, Bucky can no longer extricate himself from the troubling gift, irrespective of his best attempts at renouncing it. Unwittingly and unwillingly, he becomes enmeshed in a dangerous race to get "the product" to the street and make fortunes (a thinly veiled satire of the entertainment industry). Ironically, the product turns out to be more potent than ever imagined; in fact, it is far too strong to be practical—making the whole race to secure it a dangerous farce. When they discover that their efforts to make a fortune from it were for naught, members of Happy Valley inject Bucky with the mysterious drug to keep him quiet (as a charitable alternative to murdering him).

Thinking that he would slip into a permanent stupor, "the product" unexpectedly provides the reprieve from egoic consciousness that Bucky was seeking all along. It suppresses his left-brain function, thereby bringing a blissful preverbal and prerational state to the fore of his consciousness—a development foreshadowed by Bucky's infatuation with the severely disfigured Micklewhite boy (whose presence possessed a sheer organic power matched only by the embryonic beauty of his body). Bucky spends weeks in the "deep peace" and "immense serenity" of an ineffable peak-experience. When he finally regains his speech, he sees no reason to expound on that extended transcendental experience, or the role of the wonder drug in sustaining it.

As other examples of cannabis-inspired literature, one might cite *Farewell My Lovely, The Electric Kool-Aid Acid Test, Fear and Loathing in Las Vegas, The Time of the Assassins: A Study of Rimbaud, The Savage Detectives, Wonder Boys, King Suckerman, Valis,* and *Island*. At its most expansive, that genre might include *Alice in Wonderland*, with its Hookah-Smoking Caterpillar, or even the Hobbits' particular predilection for herbs mixed with sweet-scented flowers known as "pipe-leaf" in *Lord of the Rings*. Pipe-leaf mixes are psychoactive, and in the herblore of the Shire, Longbottom Leaf, Old Toby, and Southern Star are well-recognized strains. Hobbits possess an oft-noted proclivity for smoking herbs through pipes made from clay or wood, and it was these fur-footed creatures who taught the wizard Gandalf about the pleasures and benefits of smoking. When challenged by Saruman at the White Council regarding his preference for "Halflings' leaf," Gandalf replies that Saruman would not wonder about it, if he tried the herb: "You might find that smoke blown out," counsels Gandalf, "cleared your mind of shadows within. Anyway, it gives patience, to listen to error without anger."[66]

Contemporary cannabis fiction includes *Budding Prospects: A Pastoral* and *The African Safari Papers*, works that also depict marijuana in ways that connect it to discernment and spiritual awakening. Felix Nas-myth, the narrator protagonist of *Budding Prospects*, drops out of a doc-toral program in nineteenth-century British literature. Feeling shiftless as a result, he consents to manage a large cannabis grow-operation in north-ern California for one summer during the 1980s. In return for the possibil-ity of earning a half million dollars (tax free), he oversees a three-hun-dred-acre site, but a series of fiascos gradually diminishes the crop. Forced to harvest early to avoid arrest and imprisonment, Felix and his companions escape with what remains of their efforts. Perhaps because of the agony that they endured growing it, the first sampling is a moment "as drenched in ritual as a high mass at the Vatican." Rolling the marijuana cigarette is performed with "sacerdotal solemnity," and after it is passed around three times, Felix raises himself from his chair, and "astral specks and phantom amoebae floating unchecked" through his vision, he de-clares simply: "It's ready."[67]

Although he is slow to realize it, the irreverent and troubled protago-nist of *The African Safari Papers*, Richard Clark, finds expanded percep-tion through his experiments with cannabis, as well. When his family flies to Nairobi for a safari vacation, Richard feels compelled to travel to Kenya with an assortment of cannabis products (Humboldt County bud, vials of hash oil, and Lebanese hash). Admittedly a thoroughly unlikable chap, at Lake Baringo Camp this nineteen-year-old nevertheless smokes four bowls from his stash and falls into rapture at the beauty surrounding him. Unable to articulate that unexpected elation, it occurs to him that words have "a way of destroying beauty by trying to capture it." In choosing silence, he makes way for a startling revelation that came upon him on another occasion: if "the present moment, meaning this moment right now, is real, and five seconds ago is not real, and five seconds from now is also not real" then there really is "no beginning or end, only eternity."[68] At last, he is starting to understand the power of the present moment.

In the literary examples cited above, from François Rabelais to Théo-phile Gautier, Louise May Alcott to Robert Sedlack, cannabis use is depicted from a variety of perspectives and in different contexts that link that flowering plant to peak-experiences and highlight its entheogenic qualities. These literary treatments also help to illustrate the manifold scientific, secular, medical, and recreational engagements with cannabis in the Western world from the Renaissance until our own time (when counter values regarding the medical efficacy of marijuana are again becoming mainstream). In the brief afterword that follows, we take stock of the principal discoveries made during our spiritual exploration of cannabis in world culture, and expound upon the rationale for undertaking it sixteen years into the twenty-first century.

AFTERWORD

Fierce Bliss

In this modest study, meant to be suggestive rather than comprehensive, we have explored the manifold ways in which human beings have engaged with cannabis across time and culture. Due to its psychoactive properties, to its effectiveness as a healing agent, and to its wide availability, cannabis found a notable place in spiritual and curative traditions in Asia, the Middle East, and Africa over thousands of years. In our own time, we are seeing a revival of secular, scientific, medical, and psychological experimentations with cannabis in the United States, the Netherlands, Uruguay, and elsewhere. These developments further substantiate the value of marijuana as a safe medication and potential agent of personal transformation. After all, the search for spiritual awakening and physical healing are not two endeavors; the quest for one leads to the other. Shaman-healers and magician-alchemists understood this important truth long before the advent of record keeping, though Western medical science is just rediscovering it.

Be that as it may, I hope that readers will not misconstrue my intentions in writing this book. I do not advocate for religious or medical experimentations with cannabis in places where the plant is not yet decriminalized or legalized, but believe the day will come when more people will insist on keeping those important avenues of discovery and healing open. I clearly recognize the benefits that legal medical marijuana brings every day to children and adults suffering from maladies for which it is an effective natural treatment or curative. Leading states such as California and Colorado now permit the sale of a wide range of cannabis products (from oils to edibles, flowers to tinctures) for the focused treatment of a variety of physical and mental illnesses—sometimes without any tetrahydrocannabinol (THC) "high" whatsoever. Moreover, the fact that marijuana may be used intentionally as a mild psychoactive aid in meditation, prayer, or other concentrated religious activities adds urgency to the need for cannabis reform in the United States, and around the world.

Therefore, despite misgivings concerning the wisdom of writing about cannabis when it remains a controlled substance in many American states (and countries around the globe), the opportunity to advocate for cannabis as one of many vehicles for expanded perception propelled me onward. Considering the sea-change in public opinion in recent years favoring legalization, it seems especially urgent to call attention to how cannabis opens the door to peak-experiences in some individuals. With right practice and right intention (sustained by concentrated devotional activities such as meditation and contemplative prayer), those momentary openings may increase in frequency and duration. When the mind becomes more willing to settle into the beauty of the present moment, which may mean lingering over a single flower or leaf fluttering in the wind, a new mode of existence comes forth that leads to direct experiential understanding of the fundamentally nondual nature of reality.

If such is the case, as the proceeding chapters indicate, then the criminalization of cannabis that I witnessed growing up in the United States during the 1980s and 1990s is hard to justify. During those two decades particularly, cannabis was vilified as a "gateway drug" that led to the abuse of far more powerful substances, such as heroin or phencyclidine (PCP). On television, "public service" messages assured us that marijuana produced sloth and apathy in teenagers—or even fried their young brains like eggs on a hot skillet. So misguided was public concern about cannabis that this rather lovely flowering plant was judged a menace to the health of the individual and society writ large. Penalties for possession of small amounts of marijuana could easily result in arrest or permanent legal blemish discoverable by routine checks for jobs requiring background clearance. African Americans were inordinately targeted for possession, and cannabis arrests have filled prisons across the United States with nonviolent offenders. Some estimates suggest that blacks are still four to eight times more likely to be arrested for marijuana than whites.[1]

Given the fact that blacks and other minorities serve more time in prison for marijuana possession than whites, and consequently suffer the lingering repercussions of having a criminal record more frequently, it remains disconcerting that the United States has failed to comprehensively revisit federal cannabis law. President Barack Obama's administration has modestly relaxed enforcement of prohibitions in states with their own cannabis policies, and the Justice Department released thousands of inmates who received harsh drug sentences over the last few decades—but investigations into, and prosecutions of, violations of state and federal cannabis laws continue elsewhere (notwithstanding recent acts of presidential clemency). An ever-growing body of scientific evidence indicates a credible need to reclassify cannabis as a Schedule III substance in recognition of the lower potential of cannabis for abuse than Schedule I and II drugs, as well as new progressive medical marijuana laws in some states.

Scholars, intellectuals, doctors, and cultural critics have been pointing out for generations that the placement of cannabis on the list of Schedule I substances does not accurately represent the plant's actual psychoactive properties, nor does it account for its proven medical efficacy. Yet unreflective opposition to the decriminalization and legalization of cannabis persists. At the time of writing, the U.S. Drug Enforcement Administration (DEA) website defines Schedule I substances as those for which there is "no currently accepted medical use" and which exhibit "a high potential for abuse." Schedule I substances are treated by the legal system as "the most dangerous drugs of all the drug schedules with potentially severe psychological or physical dependence." LSD, cannabis, psilocybin, and peyote all fall into this vilified category.[2]

Schedule II substances include such highly addictive and potentially deadly agents as Dilaudid, Demerol, oxycodone, Vicodin, cocaine, methamphetamine, and methadone. Still, the DEA regards all of these restricted substances as less prone to abuse, safer, and having more medical applications than cannabis! One may conclude from such disjunctions between rhetoric and reality that Schedule I and Schedule II classifications have more to do with social morality than scientific precision. The Controlled Substances Act (CSA) schedules, which were signed into law in 1970, allow prosecution for possession of the same entheogens that were a primary means for the exploration of consciousness among members of soma and *haoma* cults, Mediterranean mystery religions, Zoroastrian priests and Islamic Sufis, and all manner of shamanistic traditions, as well as of twentieth-century religious movements such as Rastafarianism. This study, principally about cannabis, nevertheless provides historical evidence that several Schedule I substances are associated with the human quest for the divine.

While heroin, for instance, hollows inner spiritual experience and subjects users to addiction and overdose (as the current crisis in the United States shows), the unscientific inclusion of cannabis in the Schedule I category, along with entheogens such as psilocybin, may indicate a purposeful intention to limit access to peak-experiences, which make people more psychologically integrated, and therefore less susceptible to propaganda, group think, or the lures of material culture. One might imagine also that the modern pharmaceutical industry fears the effectiveness of patent-free plants like cannabis in treating many of the illnesses that synthetic medications do now—at a fraction of the cost. Whatever the case, something has gone terribly awry when millions of reasonable people understand that assertions by the U.S. Drug Enforcement Administration about cannabis are simply not true, and yet they continue to be propagated—and enforced. With more than half of all Americans now aware of the tremendous therapeutic value of medical marijuana, this may be the moment to address the politics of prohibition and institutionalized racism that led to the criminalization of cannabis in the 1930s.

We might also better appreciate the fact that changing our consciousness constitutes one of the most important relationships that human beings have with plants (consider those that give us coffee, tea, chocolate, and nicotine). Paleolithic peoples likely discovered the euphoric effects of cannabis while foraging for food; some estimates propose its continued use as a psychoactive agent for more than ten thousand years in Eurasia. [3] As we have seen, for people across the globe, hemp once provided a ready source of fiber for canvas and rope, a cellulous rich pulp for paper, a renewable fuel oil, a safe medicine, a nutritious foodstuff, a most pleasant relaxant, and a vehicle for religious experience. For such a plant to suffer criminalization, and only in the last one hundred years of human history, reflects our own unconsidered ethical biases and cultural presuppositions, rather than any botanical injuriousness. Neither sound science nor credible scholarship justifies ongoing prohibitions against cannabis when far more deadly substances such as alcohol and tobacco escape arbitrary legal bans.

Comprehensive changes in social attitudes, together with ongoing reforms of state cannabis laws, provide the long-awaited opportunity for engagement with marijuana in a more commonsensical manner than possible since the botched "war on drugs" declared by President Richard Nixon in 1971. The easing of restrictions on recreational cannabis in forward-looking American states and municipalities, together with increasing access to marijuana medicine, make possible positive psychological explorations of consciousness (including the cultivation of peak-experiences). Cannabis also holds considerable potential as a part of therapeutic regimens for depression, trauma, anxiety, and addictive disorders (such as alcoholism). Furthermore, its perennial consumption by artists and other creative individuals means a chance for more people to take advantage of the consciousness boost that the jazz improviser has valued for generations.

Meditation and other concentrated activities (dancing, praying, recitation, and mantra) have opened the door to peak-experiences for millennia, and they are all techniques of ecstasy practiced by humans since the Early Stone Age. Today, ongoing clinical studies of psychedelics at Johns Hopkins University, New York University, University of New Mexico, and other major research centers shows that two-thirds of all participants, from whom self-transcendent experiences were elicited, ranked them among the top-five most meaningful events in their entire lives.[4] The experiential components of mystical experience may be summarized at this point in our investigation: a sense of unity felt inwardly or outwardly, the transcendence of time and space, a feeling of sacredness and deeply felt positive mood, unitive knowledge, and a sense of ineffability (associated with the limitations of ratiocination and language). Peak-experiences occurred more often in research subjects prone to meditative absorption, or who openly welcomed new adventures, but they also appeared spontaneously—triggered by grief, trauma, or profound life transitions.[5] For this reason, they may be an important evolutionary psychological coping mechanism.

Plants like cannabis are nature's alchemists; they borrow our minds and bodies to disperse their seed far and wide via our two-legged (and now mechanized) locomotion. Cannabis evolved at great metabolic expense to secrete the sticky THC-rich resin, which ensures its ongoing cultivation by human beings (just as other plants generate flowery substances to attract bees and effect pollination).[6] In addition, THC acts in a similar manner as cannabinoid chemicals produced naturally in the body, and it activates the cannabinoid receptors in the brain associated with cognition, memory, pleasure, dexterity, and the awareness of time. The body's endocannabinoid system plays a significant role in perception, and the sense of elation that people experience after the activation of their THC cannabinoid receptors points to a distinctive state of consciousness, which a variety of religious and spiritual traditions (including Shaivism, Sufism, and Rastafarianism) value highly as part of ritual observance.

One naturally occurring endocannabinoid has been dubbed "anandamide" (after the Hindu term for "bliss"), and it generates psychoactive effects similar to those of marijuana: a sense of elation, transcendence, and contact with the divine.[7] As noted earlier, naturally occurring mystical experiences and those induced by chemicals are phenomenologically indistinguishable, and scientific investigations of the endocannabinoid system in the human body lend scientific credence to that observation. Psychedelic, mystical, or transcendental experiences result from seeking the sacred by moving inward—and they are found in every culture and religion around the globe. They come in silence and are discoverable in the still center of being where ordinary perception opens to the miraculous. Words prove inadequate to the task of conveying the meaning and sense of completeness that they instill. One sees the divine in the most mundane of objects, such as the spectacular beauty of a simple beam of sunlight reflected in a piece of pewterware, which triggered the first spiritual experience of seventeenth-century German mystic Jakob Böhme.

Moments of lucidity may occur spontaneously, sitting amid nature, or during daring activities that demand incredible focus (such as that of a bobsledder swooshing down an icy track). Peak-experiences are vitally important because many people living in advanced industrial economies are suffering self-imposed existential isolation from the joy of life, as well as from more natural ways of living that acknowledge the earth (and all of creation) as the self. In our technological age of scientific exploration of the empirical world, peak-experiences offer the possibility of positive inward transformation through familiarity with states of consciousness conducive to psychological and spiritual growth that result from a vision of reality as interconnected and indestructible.[8] Because society is formed of individuals acting in relation to each other and the natural world, each inward transformation by way of peak-experience effects constructive change in the "outer" world.

If we seek a better society, one in which people live self-actualized and fulfilling lives—free of ambition, competition, fear, strife, and oppression—then we must understand that even the sincerest efforts to transform human civilization before addressing the self only projects that psychological fragmentation outward (where we observe it every day in the violence, poverty, and torment that we exact on each other and the biosphere). Given the human capacity to defile and desecrate, we should avail ourselves of all means of integration and renewal. Peak-experiences offer the possibility of living more deeply and meaningfully, yet their implications need to be worked out in relation to others. They feature prominently in this study of cannabis, culture, and world religion due to their potential to remake society—as well as the self. As more people access them through intense meditation, prayer, athletics, or mild psychoactive substances like cannabis, a much needed harmony and balance will be restored to our planet.

Serious practitioners of meditation, yoga, contemplative prayer, and other spiritual arts understand that self-transcendent moments are important openings and possess considerable healing potential, but the concentrated awareness that informs peak-experiences should be extended moment after moment. One may learn to live more fully in the Now, abiding there effortlessly, without wavering, like a rock. By contrast, most of us lead dreamy existences in which our conscious attention is dragged about from one thought, desire, or judgment to another, so that direct perception of reality becomes nearly impossible. As the oft-quoted dictum by William Blake has it: "If the doors of perception were cleansed every thing would appear to man as it is: infinite. / For man has closed himself up, till he sees all things thro' narrow chinks of his cavern."[9] Unitive experiences become impossible when the egoic thought stream commands conscious attention rather than the absolute reality of the present moment. Blake understood that ordinary perception is clouded by ratiocination and consequently undervalues, or discards altogether, the transformative potential of even brief glimpses of the divine.

Individuals open to the here-now in their daily lives have already sensed its power to radically transform perception, and the world along with it. Yet no matter how beautiful or insightful, occasional glimpses of reality are not sufficient. Peak-experiences, and the freedom from time inherent within them, should culminate in "a permanent shift in consciousness." For some, sustained awakening comes with total surrender born of intense anguish, but most people work at it, which means giving one's full attention to the present moment—not only on the meditation cushion—but while engaged in all daily activities. In this way, one refuses (instant after instant) to be led away by the egoic thought stream, the default object of attention that most people erroneously endow with selfhood. Eckhart Tolle observes that the beginning of the process of "waking up" takes place with the apprehension of the habitual tendency of the mind to find the Now inadequate:

> You will observe that the future is usually imagined as either better or worse than the present. If the imagined future is better, it gives you hope or pleasurable anticipation. If it is worse, it creates anxiety. Both are illusory. Through self-observation, more *presence* comes into your life automatically. The moment you realize you are not present, you *are* present. Whenever you are able to observe your mind, you are no longer trapped in it. Another factor has come in, something that is not of the mind: the witnessing presence. [10]

We understand from this passage the basic technique of cultivating an enduring revolution in consciousness: constantly returning the mind to a state of heightened attentive awareness. Realization emerges from concentrated attention, from presence, and therefore when performed single-mindedly otherwise unremarkable daily activities (such as brushing one's teeth, taking out the trash, or driving a car) become gateways to religious experience and self-actualized living. This movement toward reverence constitutes an affirmative recognition that all life is connected on a most elemental level.

Accessing transcendental states of consciousness fundamentally transforms one's understanding of the natural world and one's place in it, regardless of whether they are evoked through intense travail, rigorous religious practice, or the ingestion of chemical agents. Peak-experiences remain essential to the advancement of the human quest for wholeness, wellness, and meaning. As Albert Einstein understood and endeavored to remind others:

The most beautiful emotion that we can experience is the mystical. It is the power of all true art and science. Those to whom this emotion is a stranger, who can no longer wonder and stand rapt in awe, are as good as dead. To know that what is impenetrable to us really exists, manifesting itself as the highest wisdom and the most radiant beauty, which our dull faculties can comprehend only in their most primitive forms—this knowledge, this feeling, is at the center of true religiousness. In this sense, and in this sense only, I belong to the rank of devoutly religious men. [11]

Here, the celebrated physicist gives voice to the power of peak-experiences, and he observes that perception of the essential dimension to which they open toward too often goes unnoticed, unappreciated, or undervalued. Moreover, the frequency with which he experiences visitations of grace suggests that entheogens are not necessary to spiritual realization—far from it.

Cannabis alone cannot bring about enlightenment—any more than concentrated attention of the kind that produces peak-experiences could suddenly transform one into an Olympic athlete or Blue Angels stunt pilot (without those skill sets in place). Even so, the religious use of plants to change consciousness precedes ancient Vedic soma rites, and plants such as psilocybin mushrooms, peyote, and marijuana have a long record of assisting people in accessing the divine. When combined with spiritual discipline, cannabis promotes spacious awareness of the contents of the mind, and simultaneously the goings-on in the "outer" world, when used with proper intention and as part of regular practice.

While not a spiritual or medical panacea, cannabis does offer access to greater imagination and creativity, heightened perspective and insight, and deeper levels of thought. What Andrew Weil terms "stoned thinking" relies on intuition *and* intellect, accepts the ambivalent nature of things, and remains open to the experience of infinity in its positive aspect (as unitive consciousness, which is the precise goal of all religions and philosophies of mind development). This mode of cognition is the mirror opposite of ordinary (or straight) thinking characterized by a heavy reliance on categorization and prejudgment, attention to outward materialistic forms, the perception of differences rather than similarities, and a tendency toward negative thought patterns. [12]

The exponential emergence of unitive consciousness through peak-experiences presents an important opportunity to create enduring positive social change through self-transformation. This is "fierce bliss," a chapter phrase meant to evoke the spiritual warriors who combat ignorance and act in response to oppression and social injustice: Siddhārtha Gautama, Mahatma Gandhi, Malcolm X, Bob Marley, and so many others like them. Fierce bliss stands for the determination to awaken to the recognition that we are one—and to start living that way. It is the creed of Sādhus, Sufis, and Rastafarians who wide-eyed challenge the dominant materialistic values of modernity along with its competition, violence, and class warfare.

Fierce bliss is the light that rouses one to action—for if there is no justice, there can be no peace. It compelled Native American shamans to reinvigorate a vanishing people wracked by war and plagues brought by Europeans. Fierce bliss drove Mother Teresa to the slums of India to care for the utterly divested, and it pushed Martin Luther King, Jr., to organize nonviolent protest marches against racial segregation. Fierce bliss fires the passion of environmentalists battling to preserve trees in old growth forests by refusing to come down from their branches, the tireless campaigner for legal medical marijuana to treat children with epilepsy, the advocate for same-sex marriage and gender equality under the law, and the Rasta speaking "dread" truth to power. Fierce bliss is ecstasy made manifest in the world.

NOTES

INTRODUCTION

1. William A. Richards, *Sacred Knowledge: Psychedelics and Religious Experiences* (New York: Columbia University Press, 2015), 23.

2. Wendy Chapkis and Richard J. Webb, *Dying to Get High: Marijuana as Medicine* (New York: New York University Press, 2008), 116.

3. Abraham Maslow, *Religions, Values, and Peak-Experiences* (Columbus: Ohio State University Press, 1964), 60–61.

4. Abraham Maslow, "Religious Aspects of Peak-Experiences," in *Personality and Religion: The Role of Religion in Personality Development*, ed. William Sadler (London: SCM Press, 1970), 174–77.

5. William Blake, *The Complete Poetry and Prose of William Blake*, ed. David Erdman (Princeton, NJ: Princeton University Press, 1991), 247.

6. Maslow, *Religions, Values, and Peak-Experiences*, 72.

7. Ibid., 64.

8. Ibid., 65.

9. John 3:3.

10. Maslow, *Religions, Values, and Peak-Experiences*, 68.

11. Daisetsu Teitaro Suzuki, *Selected Works of D. T. Suzuki, Volume I: Zen* (Berkeley: University of California Press, 2014), 82.

12. Maslow, *Religions, Values, and Peak-Experiences*, 59–60.

13. Ibid., 67.

14. David Watts, *The Psychedelic Experience: A Sociological Study* (Beverly Hills: Sage, 1971), 56–58.

15. Martin Booth, *Cannabis: A History* (New York: Picador, 2005), 13–14.

16. Ibid., 368.

I. VEDĀNTA, SĀDHU PRIESTS, AND THE "LORD OF BHANG"

1. Andrew Robinson, *India: A Short History* (London: Thames and Hudson, 2014), 11–12.

2. John Keay, *India: A History* (New York: HarperCollins, 2001), xxiv–xxvi.

3. Robinson, *India*, 35.

4. Keay, *India*, 4–5.

5. Ibid., 13–14.

6. Robinson, *India*, 36–37.

7. Raj Pruthi, *Vedic Civilization* (Delhi: Discovery Publishing, 2004), 285.

8. Robinson, *India*, 44–45.

9. Christian Rätsch, *Marijuana Medicine: A World Tour of the Healing and Visionary Powers of Cannabis* (Rochester, NY: Healing Arts Press, 2001), 15.

10. William A. Richards, *Sacred Knowledge: Psychedelics and Religious Experiences* (New York: Columbia University Press, 2015), 145.

11. Terence McKenna, *The Food of the Gods* (New York: Bantam, 1992), 7.

12. Robinson, *India*, 51–53.

13. David R. Kingsley, *Hinduism: A Cultural Perspective* (Englewood Cliffs, NJ: Prentice Hall, 1982), 11.

14. David Frawley, *The Rig Veda and the History of India* (New Delhi: Aditya Prakashan, 2001), 316–17.

15. Robinson, *India*, 53–54.

16. Ibid., 54.

17. Wendy Doniger, *The Rig Veda: An Anthology* (New York: Penguin, 1981), 134–35.

18. Franklin Edgerton, *The Beginnings of Indian Philosophy: Selections from the* Rig Veda, Atharva Veda, Upanishads, *and* Mahābhārata (Cambridge, MA: Harvard University Press, 1965), 55.

19. Michael Harner, *Hallucinogens and Shamanism* (Oxford: Oxford University Press, 1973), xi.

20. Frawley, *The Rig Veda and the History of India*, 163–66.

21. Ibid., 176–77.

22. Ralph T. H. Griffith and M. L. Abhimanyu, *Hymns of the Atharva-Veda: Volume One* (Varanasi: Master Khelari Lal & Sons, 1962), 44–46.

23. Ibid., 74.

24. Rätsch, *Marijuana Medicine*, 32.

25. S. Mahdihassan, "The Important Vedic Grasses," *Indian Journal of History of Science* 22.4 (1987): 286–91.

26. Robert Clarke and Mark Merlin, *Cannabis: Evolution and Ethnobotany* (Berkeley: University of California Press, 2013), 224–25.

27. Gavin Flood, *An Introduction to Hinduism* (Cambridge, UK: Cambridge University Press, 1996), 43–44.

28. Thomas J. Hopkins, *The Hindu Religious Tradition* (Encino, TX: Dickenson Publishing, 1971), 36–37.

29. Mircea Eliade, *A History of Religious Ideas: From Gautama Buddha to the Triumph of Christianity* (Chicago: University of Chicago Press, 1982), 45–46.

30. Eknath Easwaran, *Three Upanishads: Īshā, Māndūkya, & Shvetāshvatara* (Berkeley, CA: Blue Mountain Center, 1973), 57.

31. Eliade, *A History of Religious Ideas*, 46.

32. Edgerton, *The Beginnings of Indian Philosophy*, 46.

33. Easwaran, *Three Upanishads*, 167.

34. Eliade, *A History of Religious Ideas*, 241.

35. R. C. Zaehner, *Hindu Scriptures* (London: Everyman, 1966), 129–30.

36. Gavin Flood, ed., *The Bhagavad Gita* (New York: Norton, 2015), 47.

37. Eliade, *A History of Religious Ideas*, 70.

38. Shree Purohit and William Butler Yeats, *The Ten Principal Upanishads* (London: Faber & Faber, 1937), 33.

39. Ralph T. H. Griffith, *Rig Veda* (Benares, India: E. J. Lazarus & Co., 1896), 582.

40. Robinson, *India*, 71–72.

41. Ibid., 71.

42. James Fisher, "Cannabis in Nepal: An Overview," in *Cannabis and Culture*, ed. Vera Rubin (Paris: Mouton, 1975), 250.

43. Ibid., 250–52.

44. Stanislav Grof, "Psychedelic Research: Past, Present, and Future," in *Seeking the Sacred with Psychoactive Substances: Chemical Paths to Spirituality and to God*, ed. J. Harold Ellens (Santa Barbara, CA: Praeger, 2014), 292.

45. Khwaja A. Hasan, "Social Aspects of the Use of Cannabis in India," in *Cannabis and Culture*, ed. Vera Rubin (Paris: Mouton, 1975), 234–35.

2. SHAMANS, SUFIS, AND THE "GREEN MAN"

1. Michael Pollan, *Cannabis, Forgetting, and the Botany of Desire* (Berkeley, CA: Doreen B. Townsend Center for the Humanities, 2004), 4–5.

2. Richard Foltz, *Religions of Iran: From Prehistory to the Present* (London: One World, 2013), 11.

3. Ibid., 15.

4. Ibid., 16.

5. Edwin Bryant, *The Quest for the Origins of Vedic Culture: The Indo-Aryan Migration Debate* (Oxford: Oxford University Press, 2001), 130–31.

6. Foltz, *Religions of Iran*, 33–35.

7. Mary Boyce, *Zoroastrians: Their Religious Beliefs and Practices* (London: Routledge, 2002), 28.

8. Ibid., 29.

9. Foltz, *Religions of Iran*, 39–41.

10. Carl Ruck, Mark Hoffman, and José Celdrán, *Mushrooms, Myth, and Mithras: The Drug Cult that Civilized Europe* (San Francisco: City Lights Bookstore, 2011), 42.

11. Ansley Hamid, *The Ganja Complex: Rastafari and Marijuana* (New York: Lexington, 2002), xxxi.

12. Mircea Eliade, *Shamanism: Archaic Techniques of Ecstasy* (Princeton, NJ: Princeton University Press, 1964), 399–400.

13. Foltz, *Religions of Iran*, xii–xiii.

14. Ruck, Hoffman, and Celdrán, *Mushrooms, Myth, and Mithras*, 10–12.

15. Marvin W. Meyer, *The Ancient Mysteries: A Sourcebook* (San Francisco: Harper & Row, 1987), 199–200.

16. Ibid., 216.

17. Ibid., 211.

18. Ruck, Hoffman, and Celdrán, *Mushrooms, Myth, and Mithras*, 34–37.

19. Michael Cook, *The New Cambridge History of Islam: Volume One* (Cambridge, UK: Cambridge University Press, 2010), 161–63.

20. Molefi Kete Asante, *The History of Africa: The Quest for Eternal Harmony* (New York: Routledge, 2007), 210–11.

21. Cook, *The New Cambridge History of Islam*, 200.

22. Milad Milani, *Sufism in the Secret History of Persia* (Durham, NC: Acumen, 2013), 8–10.

23. Foltz, *Religions of Iran*, 182–83.

24. Binyamin Abrahamov, *Ibn al-'Arabi and the Sufis* (Oxford: Anqa Publishing, 2014), 3.

25. Saeko Yazaki, *Islamic Mysticism and Abū Ṭālib Al-Makkī: The Role of the Heart* (New York: Routledge, 2013), 71.

26. Nicholas Heer, trans., *Three Early Sufi Texts: A Treatise on the Heart, Stations of the Righteous, The Humble Submission of Those Aspiring* (Louisville, KY: Fons Vitae, 2009), 125–34.

27. Ibid., 135–58.

28. Claude Field, trans., *The Alchemy of Happiness by Al Ghazzali* (New York: Cosimo, 2005), 41.

29. Ibid., 44.

30. Ibid., 44.

31. Ibid., 60.

32. Alan Watts, *The Joyous Cosmology: Adventures in the Chemistry of Consciousness* (New York: New World, 2013), 15.

33. Ibid., 88.

34. Ahmed M. Khalifa, "Traditional Patterns of Hashish Use in Egypt," in *Cannabis and Culture*, ed. Vera Rubin (Paris: Mouton, 1975), 199.

35. John Renard, *Historical Dictionary of Sufism* (Toronto: Scarecrow, 2005), 97.

36. Peter Lamborn Wilson, *Scandal: Essays in Islamic Heresy* (Brooklyn, NY: Autonomedia, 1988), 213.

37. Robert Clarke and Mark Merlin, *Cannabis: Evolution and Ethnobotany* (Berkeley: University of California Press, 2013), 233.

38. Martin Booth, *Cannabis: A History* (New York: Picador, 2005), 50.

39. Jean-Louis Michon and David Streight, trans., *Two Treatises on the Oneness of Existence by the Moroccan Sufi Ahmad ibn 'Ajiba* (Cambridge, UK: Archetype, 2010), 37.

40. Ibid., 41.

41. Rumi, *The Masnavi: Book One*, trans. Jawid Mojaddedi (Oxford: Oxford University Press, 2004), 4.

42. Ibid., 4.

43. Booth, *Cannabis*, 70.

44. Ben Bennani, *Bread Hashish, and Moon: Four Modern Arab Poets* (Greensboro, NC: Unicorn Press, 1982), 5.

45. Franz Rosenthal, *The Herb: Hashish versus Medieval Muslim Society* (Leiden, The Netherlands: Brill, 1971), 163.

46. Ibid., 172–73.

47. Ibid., 149–50.

48. William Dalrymple, "The Renaissance of the Sultans," *New York Review of Books*, June 25, 2015. http://www.nybooks.com/articles/archives/2015/jun/25/renaissance-sultans/.

49. Richard Maxwell Eaton, *The Sufis of Bijapur, 1300–1700: Social Roles of Sufis in Medieval India* (Princeton, NJ: Princeton University Press, 2015), 257–58.

50. Shunryu Suzuki, *Zen Mind, Beginners Mind* (New York: Weatherhill, 1995), 7.

3. CHINESE PHARMACOPOEIA AND THE GOLDEN FLOWER

1. Robert Clarke and Mark Merlin, *Cannabis: Evolution and Ethnobotany* (Berkeley: University of California Press, 2013), 200.

2. *Book of Documents* (尚書), *Book of Changes* (易經), *Spring and Autumn Annals* (春秋), *Book of Rites* (禮記), and *Classic of Poetry* (詩經).

3. Wing-Tsit Chan, *A Source Book in Chinese Philosophy* (Princeton, NJ: Princeton University Press, 1963), 39.

4. Stephen Owen, "Foreword," in *The Book of Songs* (New York: Grove, 1996), xii–xxv.

5. Chan, *A Source Book in Chinese Philosophy*, 4.

6. Arthur Waley, trans., *The Book of Songs* (New York: Grove, 1996), 80.

7. Waley, *The Book of Songs*, 212.

8. Clarke and Merlin, *Cannabis*, 201.

9. Liao Yuqun, *Traditional Chinese Medicine* (Cambridge, UK: Cambridge University Press, 2011), 1.

10. Shou-zhong Yang, *The Divine Farmer's Materia Medica: A Translation of the Shen Nong Ben Cao Jing* (Boulder, CO: Blue Poppy Press, 2007), 148.

11. Ibid., 148.

12. Robert Svoboda and Arnie Lade, *Tao and Dharma: Chinese Medicine and Ayurveda* (Twin Lakes, WI: Lotus Press, 1995), 129.

13. Christian Rätsch, *Marijuana Medicine: A World Tour of the Healing and Visionary Powers of Cannabis* (Rochester, NY: Healing Arts Press, 2001), 4.

14. Yuqun, *Traditional Chinese Medicine*, 8.

15. Svoboda and Lade, *Tao and Dharma*, 9.

16. Carlton Kendall, "Magic Herbs: The Story of Chinese Medicine," *China Journal* 16.6 (1932): 319–20.

17. Cao Xueqin, *The Story of the Stone: The Crab-Flower Club, Volume Two* (New York: Penguin, 1981), 122–23.

18. Svoboda and Lade, *Tao and Dharma*, 16–17.

19. Gabriel Stux, Brian Berman, and Bruce Pomeranz, *Basics of Acupuncture* (Berlin: Springer, 2003), 122.

20. Yuqun, *Traditional Chinese Medicine*, 49–50.

21. Kendall, "Magic Herbs," 324–26.

22. Svoboda and Lade, *Tao and Dharma*, 31.

23. Yuqun, *Traditional Chinese Medicine*, 116.

24. Ibid., 57.

25. Ibid., 61–62.

26. Ibid., 64–65.

27. Svoboda and Lade, *Tao and Dharma*, 40–41.

28. Kee Chang Huang, *The Pharmacology of Chinese Herbs* (New York: CRC Press, 1999), 135–36.

29. *Medical Plants in China: A Selection of 150 Commonly Used Species* (Manila, Philippines: World Health Organization, 1997), 121.

30. Clarke and Merlin, *Cannabis*, 219–20.

31. Gary Edson, *Mysticism and Alchemy through the Ages: The Quest for Transformation* (Jefferson, NC: McFarland, 2012), 15.

32. Stephen Mitchell, trans., *Tao Te Ching* (New York: HarperPerennial, 1998), 4–5.

33. Ibid., 15.

34. Thomas Cleary, *The Secret of the Golden Flower: The Classic Chinese Book of Life* (New York: HarperCollins, 1991), 10–11.

35. Ibid., 42.

36. Ibid., 43.

37. Mia Touw, "The Religious and Medical Uses of Cannabis in China, India, and Tibet," *Journal of Psychoactive Drugs* 13.1 (1981): 31–32.

38. Michael Aldrich, "Tantric Cannabis Use in India," *Journal of Psychedelic Drugs* 9.3 (1977): 227–28.

39. Charles D. Orzech, ed., *Esoteric Buddhism and the Tantras in East Asia* (Leiden, The Netherlands: Brill, 2011), 5–6.

40. Jamgön Mipham, *Luminous Essence: A Guide to Guhyagarbha Tantra* (Ithaca, NY: Snow Lion, 2009), 84.

41. Anil Kumar Sarkar, *Mysteries of Vajrayana Buddhism: From Atisha to Dalai Lama* (New Delhi, India: South Asian, 1993), 40–41.

42. Vesna A. Wallace, *The Inner Kālacakratantra: A Buddhist Tantric View of the Individual* (Oxford: Oxford University Press, 2001), 49–50.

43. Mipham, *Luminous Essence*, 51.

44. Ibid., 51.

45. Ibid., 55.

4. DAGGA CULTS, COPTIC CHURCHES, AND THE RASTAFARI

1. Molefi Kete Asante, *The History of Africa: The Quest for Eternal Harmony* (New York: Routledge, 2007), 12–13.

2. Ibid., 19.

3. Ibid., 24.

4. Ibid., 29–30.

5. David Chidester, *Wild Religion: Tracking the Sacred in South Africa* (Berkeley: University of California Press, 2012), 157–58.

6. Ibid., 163–64.

7. Asante, *The History of Africa*, 31.

8. Ibid., 30.

9. Christian Rätsch, *Marijuana Medicine: A World Tour of the Healing and Visionary Powers of Cannabis* (Rochester, NY: Healing Arts Press, 2001), 86.

10. Ibid., 86–87.

11. Asante, *The History of Africa*, 209.

12. Robert Tignor, *Egypt: A Short History* (Princeton, NJ: Princeton University Press, 2010), 107.

13. James M. Robinson, ed., *Nag Hammadi Library in English* (Leiden, The Netherlands: Brill, 1990), 2–3.

14. Ibid., 297–98.

15. Ibid., 525–26.

16. Tignor, *Egypt*, 115–18.

17. Ansley Hamid, *The Ganja Complex: Rastafari and Marijuana* (Lanham, MD: Lexington, 2002), xxxii–xxxiii.

18. Franz Rosenthal, *The Herb: Hashish versus Medieval Muslim Society* (Leiden, The Netherlands: Brill, 1971), 25.

19. Ahmed M. Khalifa, "Traditional Patterns of Hashish Use in Egypt," in *Cannabis and Culture*, ed. Vera Rubin (Paris: Mouton, 1975), 199.

20. Rosenthal, *The Herb*, 56–57.

21. Rätsch, *Marijuana Medicine*, 129.

22. Abayomi Sofowora, *Medical Plants and Traditional Medicine in Africa* (New York: John Wiley and Sons, 1982), 32.

23. Gregory Adibe, *Igbo Mysticism: The Power of Igbo Traditional Religion and Society* (Onitsha: Adibe, 2008), 231–38.

24. Ibid., 105.

25. Brian M. Du Toit, "Dagga: The History and Ethnographic Setting of Cannabis Sativa in Southern Africa," in *Cannabis and Culture*, ed. Vera Rubin (Paris: Mouton, 1975): 81.

26. Rätsch, *Marijuana Medicine*, 127–28.

27. Ibid., 128–29.

28. E. M. Shaw, *The Hottentots* (Capetown: South Africa Museum, 1972), 2–10.

29. Ibid., 11.

30. Asante, *The History of Africa*, 194–95.

31. Ibid., 191–92.

32. Ibid., 197–98.

33. Ibid., 199.

34. Ibid., 200–1.

35. Rätsch, *Marijuana Medicine*, 129–30.

36. Barry S. Hewlett, "Introduction," in *Hunter-Gatherers of the Congo Basin: Cultures, Histories, and Biology of African Pygmies* (London: Transaction, 2014), xxi–xxiii.

37. Serge Bahuchet, "Cultural Diversity of African Pygmies," in *Hunter-Gatherers of the Congo Basin: Cultures, Histories, and Biology of African Pygmies*, ed. Barry S. Hewlett (London: Transaction, 2014), 12.

38. Ibid., 9–11.

39. Rätsch, *Marijuana Medicine*, 127.

40. Du Toit, "Dagga," 102–4.

41. Susanne Fürniss, "Diversity in Pygmy Music," in *Hunter-Gatherers of the Congo Basin: Cultures, Histories, and Biology of African Pygmies*, ed. Barry S. Hewlett (London: Transaction, 2014), 209.

42. Ibid., 210–11.

43. Robert E. Moïse, "Do Pygmies Have a History? Revisited: The Autochthonous Tradition in the History of Equatorial Africa," in *Hunter-Gatherers of the Congo Basin: Cultures, Histories, and Biology of African Pygmies*, ed. Barry S. Hewlett (London: Transaction, 2014), 89.

44. Augustus Henry Keane, *South Africa* (London: Edward Stanford, 1904), 119.

45. Elisée Reclus, *The Earth and Its Inhabitants*: *West Africa* (New York: Appleton, 1892), 488–89.

46. Rätsch, *Marijuana Medicine*, 129.

47. Jacob K. Olupona, *African Religions: A Very Short Introduction* (Oxford: Oxford University Press, 2014), 11–17.

48. Ibid., 5.

49. Edward Bynum, *The African Unconscious: Roots of Ancient Mysticism and Modern Psychology* (New York: Teachers College Press, 1999), 184.

50. Ibid., 185.

51. Ibid., 203.

52. Asante, *The History of Africa*, 93–94.

53. Ibid., 91.

54. Ibid., 102–3.

55. Hamid, *The Ganja Complex*, xxxiii.

56. Asante, *The History of Africa*, 222–25.

57. Robert Montgomery Martin, *Statistics of the Colonies of the British Empire* (London: W. H. Allen & Co., 1839), 7–8.

58. David Deirdre, *Rule Britannia: Women, Empire, and Victorian Writing* (Ithaca, NY: Cornell University Press, 1995), 103.

59. Ennis Edmonds, *Rastafari: A Very Short Introduction* (Oxford: Oxford University Press, 2012), 1–2.

60. Hamid, *The Ganja Complex*, 77.

61. Edmonds, *Rastafari*, 6.

62. Hamid, *The Ganja Complex*, 77–78.

63. Ibid., 87.

64. Ibid., 89.

65. Edmonds, *Rastafari*, 15.

66. Rupert Lewis, "Marcus Garvey and the Early Rastafarians," in *Rastafari: A Universal Philosophy in the Third Millennium*, ed. Werner Zips (Kingston, Jamaica: Ian Randle, 2006), 50–51.

67. Edmonds, *Rastafari*, 52–53.

68. Stephen Mitchell, *The Enlightened Mind: An Anthology of Sacred Prose* (New York: HarperCollins, 1991), 114.

69. Lambros Comitas, "The Social Nexus of Ganja in Jamaica," in *Cannabis and Culture*, ed. Vera Rubin (Paris: Mouton, 1975): 128–30.

70. Rätsch, *Marijuana Medicine*, 138–39.

71. Ibid., 138.

72. Martin Booth, *Cannabis: A History* (New York: Picador, 2005), 317.

73. Edmonds, *Rastafari*, 48–49.

74. Ibid.,, 45.

75. Michael Barnett, *Rastafari in the New Millennium: A Rastafari Reader* (Syracuse, NY: Syracuse University Press, 2012), 69–79.

5. PEAK-EXPERIENCES AND THE INEFFABLE

1. William A. Richards, *Sacred Knowledge: Psychedelics and Religious Experiences* (New York: Columbia University Press, 2015), 16–17.

2. Ibid., 17.

3. Ibid., 207–8.

4. Abraham Maslow, "Religious Aspects of Peak-Experiences," in *Personality and Religion: The Role of Religion in Personality Development*, ed. William Sadler (London: SCM Press, 1970), 169–70.

5. Kenneth Kraft, *Eloquent Zen: Daitō and Early Japanese Zen* (Honolulu: University of Hawaii Press, 1997), 93.

6. Eckhart Tolle, *The Power of Now* (Vancouver: Namaste, 2004), 4–5.

7. Ibid., 52.

8. Abraham Maslow, *Religions, Values, and Peak-Experiences* (Columbus: Ohio State University Press, 1964), 64–65.

9. Maslow, "Religious Aspects of Peak-Experiences," 174–77.

10. Ibid., 178.

11. Maslow, *Religions, Values, and Peak-Experiences*, 19–21.

12. Robert Jesse and Roland Griffiths, "Psilocybin Research at Johns Hopkins: A 2014 Report," in *Seeking the Sacred with Psychoactive Substances: Chemical Paths to Spirituality and to God*, ed. J. Harold Ellens (Santa Barbara, CA: Praeger, 2014), 34–38.

13. Maslow, "Religious Aspects of Peak-Experiences," 28–29.

14. David Steindl-Rast, "Psychoactive Substances and Sacred Values: Reconsidering Abraham Maslow's Discoveries," in *Seeking the Sacred with Psychoactive Substances: Chemical Paths to Spirituality and to God*, ed. J. Harold Ellens (Santa Barbara, CA: Praeger, 2014), 384–86.

15. Alan Watts, *The Art of Contemplation* (New York: Pantheon, 1972), 1.

16. Richards, *Sacred Knowledge*, 208.

17. Hugh Bowden, *Mystery Cults of the Ancient World* (Princeton, NJ: Princeton University Press, 2010), 9–11.

18. Mircea Eliade, *A History of Religious Ideas: From Gautama Buddha to the Triumph of Christianity* (Chicago: University of Chicago Press, 1982), 280.

19. Bowden, *Mystery Cults of the Ancient World*, 27–28.

20. Ibid., 37–38.

21. Carl Ruck, "The Greek Hero and the Herbal Fantasies: Entheogenic Theriomorphism and the Hero Myth," in *Seeking the Sacred with Psychoactive Substances: Chemical Paths to Spirituality and to God*, ed. J. Harold Ellens (Santa Barbara, CA: Praeger, 2014), 67.

22. Bowden, *Mystery Cults of the Ancient World*, 40.

23. Theodore Brunner, "Marijuana in Ancient Greece and Rome? The Literary Evidence," *Bulletin of the History of Medicine* 47.4 (1973): 349.

24. Ernest L. Abel, *Marihuana: The First Twelve Thousand Years* (New York: Springer, 1980), 34–35.

25. Martin Booth, *Cannabis: A History* (New York: Picador, 2005), 31.

26. Michael A. Rinella, *Pharmakon: Plato, Drug Culture, and Identity in Ancient Athens* (Lanham, MD: Lexington Books, 2010), 76–87.

27. Booth, *Cannabis: A History*, 46.

28. Renate Rolle, *The World of the Scythians* (Berkeley: University of California Press, 1989), 91–92.

29. Ibid., 93.

30. Ibid., 21–22.

31. Ibid., 86–89.

32. Timothy Knepper, "Ineffability," in *Vocabulary for the Study of Religion*, ed. Robert Segal and Kocku von Stuckrad (Leiden, The Netherlands: Brill, 2015), 28.

33. Mircea Eliade, *Shamanism: Archaic Techniques of Ecstasy* (Princeton, NJ: Princeton University Press, 2004), 3.

34. Ibid., 4.

35. Ibid., 5–6.

36. Ibid., 96.

37. Ibid., 99.

38. Vera Rubin, "The Ganja Vision in Jamaica," in *Cannabis and Culture*, ed. Vera Rubin (Paris: Mouton, 1975), 264–65.

39. Ibid., 262–63.

40. Eliade, *Shamanism*, 298–99.

41. Ibid., 314–15.

42. Ibid., 324–29.

43. Michael Winkelman, "Shamanistic Consciousness and Human Evolution," in *Seeking the Sacred with Psychoactive Substances: Chemical Paths to Spirituality and to God*, ed. J. Harold Ellens (Santa Barbara, CA: Praeger, 2014), 130.

44. Roger Walsh, "The Religious Use of Psychedelic Experiences in Shamanism and the Question of the Value and Validity of Such Experiences," in *Seeking the Sacred with Psychoactive Substances: Chemical Paths to Spirituality and to God*, ed. J. Harold Ellens (Santa Barbara: Praeger, 2014), 169–70.

45. Roberto Mario Salmón, *Indian Revolts in Northern New Spain: A Synthesis of Resistance, 1680–1786* (Lanham, MD: University Press of America, 1991), 21–22.

46. Martin A. Lee, *Smoke Signals: A Social History of Marijuana: Medical, Recreational, and Scientific* (New York: Scribner, 2013), 38–39.

47. Roberto Williams-Garcia, "The Ritual Use of Cannabis in Mexico," in *Cannabis and Culture*, ed. Vera Rubin (Paris: Mouton, 1975), 138.

48. Ibid., 140.

49. Booth, *Cannabis*, 187.

50. James W. Herrick, *Iroquois Medical Botany* (Syracuse, NY: Syracuse University Press, 1995), 89–91.

51. Ibid., 198.

52. Anthony Wonderley, *Oneida Iroquois Folklore, Myth, and History: New York Oral Narrative from the Notes of H. E. Allen and Others* (Syracuse, NY: Syracuse University Press, 2004), 12–13.

53. Christian Rätsch, *Marijuana Medicine: A World Tour of the Healing and Visionary Powers of Cannabis* (Rochester, NY: Healing Arts Press, 2001), 144.

6. HASHISH EATERS, HOBBITS' LEAF, AND THE PANTAGRUELION

1. Mark S. Ferrara, *Palace of Ashes: China and the Decline of American Higher Education* (Baltimore: Johns Hopkins University Press, 2015), 63.

2. Ibid., 60.

3. M. A. Screech, trans., *François Rabelais: Gargantua and Pantagruel* (New York: Penguin, 2006), xxiii.

4. Ibid., xxvi.

5. Ibid., 228

6. Ibid., 246.

7. Ibid., 247.

8. A. J. Krailsheimer, *Rabelais and the Franciscans* (Oxford: Clarendon, 1963), 175.

9. François Rabelais, *Gargantua and Pantagruel* (New York: Penguin, 2006), 373.

10. Ibid., 368–70.

11. Ibid., 364–67.

12. Ibid., 372–73.

13. Edwin M. Duval, "Pantagruelism," in *The Rabelais Encyclopedia*, ed. Elizabeth Chesney Zegura (Westport, CT: Greenwood, 2004), 178–79.

14. François Rigolot, "Pantagruelion" in *The Rabelais Encyclopedia*, ed. Elizabeth Chesney Zegura (Westport, CT: Greenwood, 2004), 176–77.

15. Screech, *François Rabelais*, 606–7.

16. Ibid., 600–1.

17. Ibid., 599.

18. Ibid., 614.

19. Martin A. Lee, *Smoke Signals: A Social History of Marijuana: Medical, Recreational, and Scientific* (New York: Scribner, 2013), 28.

20. Martin Booth, *Cannabis: A History* (New York: Picador, 2005), 83–84.

21. Derek Stanford, "Introduction," in *Hashish, Wine, Opium: Théophile Gautier and Charles Baudelaire* (London: One World Classics, 2009), vii.

22. Booth, *Cannabis*, 84–85.

23. Théophile Gautier, "Hashish," in *Hashish, Wine, Opium: Théophile Gautier and Charles Baudelaire* (London: One World Classics, 2009), 57.

24. Ibid., 59.

25. Ibid., 60.

26. Théophile Gautier, "The Club of Assassins," in *Hashish, Wine, Opium: Théophile Gautier and Charles Baudelaire* (London: One World Classics, 2009), 39.

27. Charles Baudelaire, "On Wine and Hashish," in *Charles Baudelaire: Artificial Paradises*, ed. Stacy Diamond (New York: Citadel Press, 1996), 15.

28. Stanford, "Introduction," xiii.

29. Charles Baudelaire, "The Poem of Hashish," in *Charles Baudelaire: Artificial Paradises*, ed. Stacy Diamond (New York: Citadel Press, 1996), 63.

30. Ibid., 50.

31. Ibid., 51.

32. Ibid., 60.

33. Stephen Rachman, "Introduction," in *The Hasheesh Eater: Being Passages from the Life of a Pythagorean*, by Fitz Hugh Ludlow (New Brunswick, NJ: Rutgers University Press, 2006), xv–xviii.

34. Donald P. Dulchinos, *Pioneer of Inner Space: The Life of Fitz Hugh Ludlow, Hasheesh Eater* (Brooklyn, NY: Autonomedia, 1998), 59.

35. Richard Boire and Kevin Feeney, *Medical Marijuana Law* (Oakland, CA: Ronin Publishing, 2006), 15–16.

36. Dulchinos, *Pioneer of Inner Space*, 45.

37. Fitz Hugh Ludlow, *The Hasheesh Eater: Being Passages from the Life of a Pythagorean* (New Brunswick, NJ: Rutgers University Press, 2006), 171–72.

38. Ibid., 298.

39. Madeleine Stern, "Introduction," in *Louisa May Alcott Unmasked: Collected Thrillers* (Boston: Northeastern University Press, 1995), xxi.

40. Ibid., xi–xv.

41. Louisa May Alcott, "The Perilous Play," in *Louisa May Alcott Unmasked: Collected Thrillers*, edited by Madeleine Stern (Boston: Northeastern University Press, 1995), 686–87.

42. Ibid., 688–89.

43. Ibid., 690–91.

44. Ibid., 693–94.

45. Stern, "Introduction," xxiii–xv.

46. Susan Roberts, *The Magician of the Golden Dawn: The Story of Aleister Crowley* (Chicago: Contemporary Books, 1978), 3–4.

47. Ibid., 52–60.

48. Ibid., 187.

49. W. B. Yeats, *Autobiography: Consisting of Reveries over Childhood and Youth, The Trembling of the Veil, and Dramatis Personae* (New York: Macmillan, 1953), 295.

50. Shree Purohit and William Butler Yeats, *The Ten Principal Upanishads* (London: Faber and Faber, 1937), 15–16.

51. Howard Eiland, ed., "Foreword," in *On Hashish: Walter Benjamin* (Cambridge, MA: Belknap, 2006), vii.

52. Marcus Boon, "Introduction," in *On Hashish: Walter Benjamin*, ed. Howard Eiland (Cambridge, MA: Belknap, 2006), 10–11.

53. Eiland, "Foreword," xi–xii.

54. Walter Benjamin, "Protocols of Drug Experiments," in *On Hashish: Walter Benjamin*, ed. Howard Eiland (Cambridge, MA: Belknap, 2006), 50–53.

55. Howard Eiland and Michael Jennings, *Walter Benjamin: A Critical Life* (Cambridge, MA: Belknap Press, 2014), 675.

56. Allen Ginsberg, "First Manifesto to End the Bringdown," in *The Marihuana Papers*, edited by David Solomon (Indianapolis: Bobbs-Merrill, 1966), 184–85.

57. Ibid., 190–96.

58. Ibid., 196–97.

59. Ibid., 199–200.

60. Joan Didion, *Slouching toward Bethlehem* (New York: Farrar, Straus & Giroux, 1968), 84–87.

61. Ibid., 97–102.

62. Ibid., 112–13.

63. Ibid., 127–28.

64. Paul Bowles, "The Story of Lahcen and Idir," in *The Marihuana Papers*, ed. David Solomon (Indianapolis: Bobbs-Merrill, 1966), 169–70.

65. Terry Southern, "Red Dirt Marihuana," in *The Marihuana Papers*, edited by David Solomon (Indianapolis: Bobbs-Merrill, 1966), 178–82.

66. J. R. R. Tolkien, *Unfinished Tales of Númenor and Middle-Earth* (New York: Ballantine, 1980), 362–66.

67. T. C. Boyle, *Budding Prospects: A Pastoral* (New York: Viking, 1984), 304–5.

68. Robert Sedlack, *The African Safari Papers* (Woodstock, NY: Overlook Press, 2003), 85, 283.

AFTERWORD

1. Ian Urbina, "Blacks Are Singled Out for Marijuana Arrests, Federal Data Suggests," *New York Times*, June 3, 2013. http://www.nytimes.com/2013/06/04/us/marijuana-arrests-four-times-as-likely-for-blacks.html.

2. DEA, Drug Scheduling at: http://www.dea.gov/druginfo/ds.shtml.

3. Robert Clarke and Mark Merlin, *Cannabis: Evolution and Ethnobotany* (Berkeley: University of California Press, 2013), 213–17.

4. Michael Pollan, "The Trip Treatment," *New York Times*, February 9, 2015. http://www.newyorker.com/magazine/2015/02/09/trip-treatment.

5. David Yaden and Andrew Newberg, "A New Means for Perennial Ends: Self-Transcendent Experiences and Noninvasive Brain Stimulation," in *Seeking the Sacred with Psychoactive Substances: Chemical Paths to Spirituality and to God*, ed. J. Harold Ellens (Santa Barbara, CA: Praeger, 2014), 307.

6. Michael Pollan, *Cannabis, Forgetting, and the Botany of Desire* (Berkeley, CA: Doreen B. Townsend Center for the Humanities, 2004), 4–6.

7. Michael Winkelman, "Evolutionary Views of Entheogenic Consciousness," in *Seeking the Sacred with Psychoactive Substances: Chemical Paths to Spirituality and to God*, ed. J. Harold Ellens (Santa Barbara, CA: Praeger, 2014), 348.

8. William A. Richards, "The Rebirth of Research with Entheogens: Lessons from the Past and Hypotheses for the Future," in *Seeking the Sacred with*

Psychoactive Substances: Chemical Paths to Spirituality and to God, ed. J. Harold Ellens (Santa Barbara, CA: Praeger, 2014), 2.

9. William Blake, "The Marriage of Heaven and Hell," in *The Complete Poetry and Prose of William Blake*, edited by David Erdman (Princeton, NJ: Princeton University Press, 1991), 39.

10. Eckhart Tolle, *The Power of Now* (Vancouver: Namaste, 2004), 55.

11. Yaden and Newberg, "A New Means for Perennial Ends," 305–6.

12. Andrew Weil, *The Natural Mind: A New Way to Look at Drugs and the Higher Consciousness* (New York: Houghton Mifflin, 1972), 149–55.

BIBLIOGRAPHY

Abel, Ernest L. *Marihuana: The First Twelve Thousand Years*. New York: Springer, 1980.

Abrahamov, Binyamin. *Ibn al-'Arabi and the Sufis*. Oxford: Anqa Publishing, 2014.

Adibe, Gregory. *Igbo Mysticism: The Power of Igbo Traditional Religion and Society*. Onitsha: Adibe, 2008.

Alcott, Louisa May. "The Perilous Play." In *Louisa May Alcott Unmasked: Collected Thrillers*, edited by Madeleine Stern, 686–94. Boston: Northeastern University Press, 1995.

Aldrich, Michael. "Tantric Cannabis Use in India." *Journal of Psychedelic Drugs* 9.3 (1977): 227–33.

Asante, Molefi Kete. *The History of Africa: The Quest for Eternal Harmony*. New York: Routledge, 2007.

Bahuchet, Serge. "Cultural Diversity of African Pygmies." In *Hunter-Gatherers of the Congo Basin: Cultures, Histories, and Biology of African Pygmies*, edited by Barry S. Hewlett, 1–29. London: Transaction, 2014.

Barnett, Michael. *Rastafari in the New Millennium: A Rastafari Reader*. Syracuse, NY: Syracuse University Press, 2012.

Baudelaire, Charles. "On Wine and Hashish." In *Charles Baudelaire: Artificial Paradises*, edited by Stacy Diamond, 3–25. New York: Citadel Press, 1996.

———. "The Poem of Hashish." In *Charles Baudelaire: Artificial Paradises*, edited by Stacy Diamond, 31–76. New York: Citadel Press, 1996.

Benjamin, Walter. "Protocols of Drug Experiments." In *On Hashish: Walter Benjamin*, edited by Howard Eiland, 17–101. Cambridge, MA: Belknap, 2006.

Bennani, Ben. *Bread Hashish, and Moon: Four Modern Arab Poets*. Greensboro, NC: Unicorn Press, 1982.

Blake, William. *The Complete Poetry and Prose of William Blake*. Edited by David Erdman. Princeton, NJ: Princeton University Press, 1991.

———. "The Marriage of Heaven and Hell." In *The Complete Poetry and Prose of William Blake*, edited by David Erdman, 33–43. Princeton, NJ: Princeton University Press, 1991.

Boire, Richard, and Kevin Feeney. *Medical Marijuana Law*. Oakland, CA: Ronin Publishing, 2006.

Boon, Marcus. "Introduction." In *On Hashish: Walter Benjamin*, edited by Howard Eiland, 1–12. Cambridge, MA: Belknap, 2006.

Booth, Martin. *Cannabis: A History*. New York: Picador, 2005.

Bowden, Hugh. *Mystery Cults of the Ancient World*. Princeton, NJ: Princeton University Press, 2010.

Bowles, Paul. "The Story of Lahcen and Idir." In *The Marihuana Papers*, edited by David Solomon, 163–70. Indianapolis: Bobbs-Merrill, 1966.

Boyce, Mary. *Zoroastrians: Their Religious Beliefs and Practices*. London: Routledge, 2002.

Boyle, T. C. *Budding Prospects: A Pastoral*. New York: Viking, 1984.

Brunner, Theodore. "Marijuana in Ancient Greece and Rome? The Literary Evidence." *Bulletin of the History of Medicine* 47.4 (1973): 344–55.

Bryant, Edwin. *The Quest for the Origins of Vedic Culture: The Indo-Aryan Migration Debate*. Oxford: Oxford University Press, 2001.

Bynum, Edward. *The African Unconscious: Roots of Ancient Mysticism and Modern Psychology*. New York: Teachers College Press, 1999.

Cao Xueqin. *The Story of the Stone: The Crab-Flower Club, Volume Two*. New York: Penguin, 1981.

Chan, Wing-Tsit. *A Source Book in Chinese Philosophy*. Princeton, NJ: Princeton University Press, 1963.

Chapkis, Wendy, and Richard J. Webb. *Dying to Get High: Marijuana as Medicine*. New York: New York University Press, 2008.

Chesney, Elizabeth A., ed. *The Rabelais Encyclopedia*. Westport, CT: Greenwood, 2004.

Chidester, David. *Wild Religion: Tracking the Sacred in South Africa*. Berkeley: University of California Press, 2012.

Clarke, Robert, and Mark Merlin. *Cannabis: Evolution and Ethnobotany*. Berkeley: University of California Press, 2013.

Cleary, Thomas. *The Secret of the Golden Flower: The Classic Chinese Book of Life*. New York: HarperCollins, 1991.

Comitas, Lambros. "The Social Nexus of Ganja in Jamaica." In *Cannabis and Culture*, edited by Vera Rubin, 119–32. Paris: Mouton, 1975.

Cook, Michael. *The New Cambridge History of Islam: Volume One*. Cambridge, UK: Cambridge University Press, 2010.

Dalrymple, William. "The Renaissance of the Sultans." *New York Review of Books*, June 25, 2015. http://www.nybooks.com/articles/archives/2015/jun/25/renaissance-sultans/.

Didion, Joan. *Slouching toward Bethlehem*. New York: Farrar, Straus & Giroux, 1968.

Deirdre, David. *Rule Britannia: Women, Empire, and Victorian Writing*. Ithaca, NY: Cornell University Press, 1995.

Doniger, Wendy. *The Rig Veda: An Anthology*. New York: Penguin, 1981.

Dulchinos, Donald P. *Pioneer of Inner Space: The Life of Fitz Hugh Ludlow, Hasheesh Eater*. Brooklyn, NY: Autonomedia, 1998.

Du Toit, Brian M. "Dagga: The History and Ethnographic Setting of Cannabis Sativa in Southern Africa." In *Cannabis and Culture*, edited by Vera Rubin, 81–116. Paris: Mouton, 1975.

———. "Man and Cannabis in Africa: A Study of Diffusion." *African Economic History* 1 (1976): 17–35.

Duval, Edwin M. "Pantagruelism." In *The Rabelais Encyclopedia*, edited by Elizabeth Chesney Zegura, 178–79. Westport, CT: Greenwood, 2004.

Easwaran, Eknath. *Three Upanishads: Īshā, Māndūkya, & Shvetāshvatara*. Berkeley, CA: Blue Mountain Center, 1973.

Eaton, Richard Maxwell. *The Sufis of Bijapur, 1300–1700: Social Roles of Sufis in Medieval India*. Princeton, NJ: Princeton University Press, 2015.

Edgerton, Franklin. *The Beginnings of Indian Philosophy: Selections from the Rig Veda, Atharva Veda, Upanishads, and Mahābhārata*. Cambridge, MA: Harvard University Press, 1965.

Edmonds, Ennis. *Rastafari: A Very Short Introduction*. Oxford: Oxford University Press, 2012.

Edson, Gary. *Mysticism and Alchemy through the Ages: The Quest for Transformation*. Jefferson, NC: McFarland, 2012.

Eiland, Howard. "Foreword." In *On Hashish: Walter Benjamin*, vii–xii. Cambridge, MA: Belknap, 2006.

Eiland, Howard, and Michael Jennings. *Walter Benjamin: A Critical Life*. Cambridge, MA: Belknap Press, 2014.

Eliade, Mircea. *Shamanism: Archaic Techniques of Ecstasy*. Princeton, NJ: Princeton University Press, 1964.

————. *A History of Religious Ideas: From Gautama Buddha to the Triumph of Christianity.* Chicago: University of Chicago Press, 1982.

Ferrara, Mark S. *Palace of Ashes: China and the Decline of American Higher Education.* Baltimore: Johns Hopkins University Press, 2015.

Field, Claude, trans. *The Alchemy of Happiness by Al Ghazzali.* New York: Cosimo, 2005.

Fisher, James. "Cannabis in Nepal: An Overview." In *Cannabis and Culture,* edited by Vera Rubin, 247–55. Paris: Mouton, 1975.

Flood, Gavin. *An Introduction to Hinduism.* Cambridge, UK: Cambridge University Press, 1996.

————, ed. *The Bhagavad Gita.* New York: Norton, 2015.

Foltz, Richard. *Religions of Iran: From Prehistory to the Present.* London: One World, 2013.

Frawley, David. *The Rig Veda and the History of India.* New Delhi: Aditya Prakashan, 2001.

Fürniss, Susanne. "Diversity in Pygmy Music." In *Hunter-Gatherers of the Congo Basin: Cultures, Histories, and Biology of African Pygmies,* edited by Barry S. Hewlett, 187–218. London: Transaction, 2014.

Gautier, Théophile. "The Club of Assassins." In *Hashish, Wine, Opium: Théophile Gautier and Charles Baudelaire,* 19–54. London: One World Classics, 2009.

————. "Hashish." In *Hashish, Wine, Opium: Théophile Gautier and Charles Baudelaire,* 55–62. London: One World Classics, 2009.

Ginsberg, Allen. "First Manifesto to End the Bringdown." In *The Marihuana Papers,* edited by David Solomon, 183–200. Indianapolis: Bobbs-Merrill, 1966.

Griffith, Ralph T. H. *Rig Veda.* Benares, India: E. J. Lazarus & Co., 1896.

Griffith, Ralph T. H., and M. L. Abhimanyu. *Hymns of the Atharva-Veda: Volume One.* Varanasi, India: Master Khelari Lal & Sons, 1962.

Grof, Stanislav. "Psychedelic Research: Past, Present, and Future." In *Seeking the Sacred with Psychoactive Substances: Chemical Paths to Spirituality and to God,* edited by J. Harold Ellens, 291–302. Santa Barbara, CA: Praeger, 2014.

Hamid, Ansley. *The Ganja Complex: Rastafari and Marijuana.* New York: Lexington, 2002.

Harner, Michael. *Hallucinogens and Shamanism.* Oxford: Oxford University Press, 1973.

Hasan, Khwaja A. "Social Aspects of the Use of Cannabis in India." In *Cannabis and Culture,* edited by Vera Rubin, 234–46. Paris: Mouton, 1975.

Heer, Nicholas, trans. *Three Early Sufi Texts: A Treatise on the Heart, Stations of the Righteous, The Humble Submission of Those Aspiring.* Louisville, KY: Fons Vitae, 2009.

Herrick, James W. *Iroquois Medical Botany.* Syracuse, NY: Syracuse University Press, 1995.

Hewlett, Barry S., ed. *Hunter-Gatherers of the Congo Basin: Cultures, Histories, and Biology of African Pygmies.* London: Transaction, 2014.

Hopkins, Thomas J. *The Hindu Religious Tradition.* Encino, TX: Dickenson Publishing, 1971.

Huang, Kee Chang. *The Pharmacology of Chinese Herbs.* New York: CRC Press, 1999.

Jesse, Robert, and Roland Griffiths. "Psilocybin Research at Johns Hopkins: A 2014 Report." In *Seeking the Sacred with Psychoactive Substances: Chemical Paths to Spirituality and to God,* edited by J. Harold Ellens, 29–43. Santa Barbara, CA: Praeger, 2014.

Keane, Augustus Henry. *South Africa.* London: Edward Stanford, 1904.

Keay, John. *India: A History.* New York: HarperCollins, 2001.

Kendall, Carlton. "Magic Herbs: The Story of Chinese Medicine." *China Journal* 16.6 (1932): 319–20.

Khalifa, Ahmed M. "Traditional Patterns of Hashish Use in Egypt." In *Cannabis and Culture,* edited by Vera Rubin, 195–205. Paris: Mouton, 1975.

Kingsley, David R. *Hinduism: A Cultural Perspective.* Englewood Cliffs, NJ: Prentice Hall, 1982.

Knepper, Timothy. "Ineffability." In *Vocabulary for the Study of Religion,* edited by Robert Segal and Kocku von Stuckrad. Leiden, The Netherlands: Brill, 2015. http://referenceworks.brillonline.com/entries/vocabulary-for-the-study-of-religion/ineffability-COM_00000347.

Kraft, Kenneth. *Eloquent Zen: Daitō and Early Japanese Zen.* Honolulu: University of Hawaii Press, 1997.

Krailsheimer, A. J. *Rabelais and the Franciscans.* Oxford: Clarendon, 1963.

Lee, Martin A. *Smoke Signals: A Social History of Marijuana: Medical, Recreational, and Scientific*. New York: Scribner, 2013.

Lewis, Rupert. "Marcus Garvey and the Early Rastafarians." In *Rastafari: A Universal Philosophy in the Third Millennium*, edited by Werner Zips, 42–58. Kingston, Jamaica: Ian Randle, 2006.

Liao Yuqun. *Traditional Chinese Medicine*. Cambridge, UK: Cambridge University Press, 2011.

Ludlow, Fitz Hugh. *The Hasheesh Eater: Being Passages from the Life of a Pythagorean*. New Brunswick, NJ: Rutgers University Press, 2006.

Mahdihassan, S. "Three Important Vedic Grasses." *Indian Journal of History of Science* 22.4 (1987): 286–91.

Martin, Robert Montgomery. *Statistics of the Colonies of the British Empire*. London: W. H. Allen & Co., 1839.

Maslow, Abraham. *Religions, Values, and Peak-Experiences*. Columbus: Ohio State University Press, 1964.

————. "Religious Aspects of Peak-Experiences." In *Personality and Religion: The Role of Religion in Personality Development*, edited by William Sadler, 168–79. London: SCM Press, 1970.

McKenna, Terence. *The Food of the Gods*. New York: Bantam, 1992.

Medical Plants in China: A Selection of 150 Commonly Used Species. Manila, Philippines: World Health Organization, 1997.

Meyer, Marvin W. *The Ancient Mysteries: A Sourcebook*. San Francisco: Harper & Row, 1987.

Michon, Jean-Louis, and David Streight, trans. *Two Treatises on the Oneness of Existence by the Moroccan Sufi Ahmad ibn 'Ajiba*. Cambridge, UK: Archetype, 2010.

Milani, Milad. *Sufism in the Secret History of Persia*. Durham, NC: Acumen, 2013.

Mipham, Jamgön. *Luminous Essence: A Guide to Guhyagarbha Tantra*. Ithaca, NY: Snow Lion, 2009.

Mitchell, Stephen. *The Enlightened Mind: An Anthology of Sacred Prose*. New York: HarperCollins, 1991.

————, trans. *Tao Te Ching*. New York: HarperPerennial, 1998.

Moïse, Robert E. "Do Pygmies Have a History: The Autochthonous Tradition in the History of Equatorial Africa." In *Hunter-Gatherers of the Congo Basin: Cultures, Histories, and Biology of African Pygmies*, edited by Barry S. Hewlett, 85–116. London: Transaction, 2014.

Olupona, Jacob K. *African Religions: A Very Short Introduction*. Oxford: Oxford University Press, 2014.

Orzech, Charles D. *Esoteric Buddhism and the Tantras in East Asia*. Leiden, The Netherlands: Brill, 2011.

Owen, Stephen. "Foreword." In *The Book of Songs*, xii–xxv. New York: Grove, 1996.

Pollan, Michael. *Cannabis, Forgetting, and the Botany of Desire*. Berkeley, CA: Doreen B. Townsend Center for the Humanities, 2004.

————. "The Trip Treatment." *New York Times*, February 9, 2015. http://www.newyorker.com/magazine/2015/02/09/trip-treatment.

Pruthi, Raj. *Vedic Civilization*. Delhi, India: Discovery Publishing, 2004.

Purohit, Shree, and William Butler Yeats. *The Ten Principal Upanishads*. London: Faber and Faber, 1937.

Rabelais, François. *Gargantua and Pantagruel*. New York: Penguin, 2006.

Rachman, Stephen. "Introduction." *The Hasheesh Eater: Being Passages from the Life of a Pythagorean*, by Fitz Hugh Ludlow, ix–xxxvi. New Brunswick, NJ: Rutgers University Press, 2006.

Rätsch, Christian. *Marijuana Medicine: A World Tour of the Healing and Visionary Powers of Cannabis*. Rochester, NY: Healing Arts Press, 2001.

Reclus, Elisée. *The Earth and Its Inhabitants: West Africa*. New York: Appleton, 1892.

Renard, John. *Historical Dictionary of Sufism*. Toronto: Scarecrow, 2005.

Richards, William A. "The Rebirth of Research with Entheogens: Lessons from the Past and Hypotheses for the Future." In *Seeking the Sacred with Psychoactive Substances: Chemical

Paths to Spirituality and to God, edited by J. Harold Ellens, 1–14. Santa Barbara, CA: Praeger, 2014.

———. *Sacred Knowledge: Psychedelics and Religious Experiences*. New York: Columbia University Press, 2015.

Rigolot, François. "Pantagruelion." In *The Rabelais Encyclopedia*, edited by Elizabeth Chesney Zegura, 176–78. Westport, CT: Greenwood, 2004.

Rinella, Michael A. *Pharmakon: Plato, Drug Culture, and Identity in Ancient Athens*. Lanham, MD: Lexington Books, 2010.

Roberts, Susan. *The Magician of the Golden Dawn: The Story of Aleister Crowley*. Chicago: Contemporary Books, 1978.

Robinson, Andrew. *India: A Short History*. London: Thames and Hudson, 2014.

Robinson, James M., ed. *Nag Hammadi Library in English*. Leiden, The Netherlands: Brill, 1990.

Rolle, Renate. *The World of the Scythians*. Berkeley: University of California Press, 1989.

Rosenthal, Franz. *The Herb: Hashish versus Medieval Muslim Society*. Leiden, The Netherlands: Brill, 1971.

Rubin, Vera. "The Ganja Vision in Jamaica." In *Cannabis and Culture*, edited by Vera Rubin, 257–66. Paris: Mouton, 1975.

Ruck, Carl. "The Greek Hero and the Herbal Fantasies: Entheogenic Theriomorphism and the Hero Myth." In *Seeking the Sacred with Psychoactive Substances: Chemical Paths to Spirituality and to God*, edited by J. Harold Ellens, 57–71. Santa Barbara, CA: Praeger, 2014.

Ruck, Carl, Mark Hoffman, and José Celdrán. *Mushrooms, Myth, and Mithras: The Drug Cult that Civilized Europe*. San Francisco: City Lights Bookstore, 2011.

Rumi. *The Masnavi: Book One*. Translated by Jawid Mojaddedi. Oxford: Oxford University Press, 2004.

Salmón, Roberto Mario. *Indian Revolts in Northern New Spain: A Synthesis of Resistance, 1680–1786*. Lanham, MD: University Press of America, 1991.

Sarkar, Anil Kumar. *Mysteries of Vajrayana Buddhism: From Atisha to Dalai Lama*. New Delhi, India: South Asian, 1993.

Screech, M. A., trans. *François Rabelais: Gargantua and Pantagruel*. New York: Penguin, 2006.

Sedlack, Robert. *The African Safari Papers*. Woodstock, NY: Overlook Press, 2003.

Shaw, E. M. *The Hottentots*. Cape Town: South Africa Museum, 1972.

Sofowora, Abayomi. *Medical Plants and Traditional Medicine in Africa*. New York: John Wiley and Sons, 1982.

Southern, Terry. "Red Dirt Marihuana." In *The Marihuana Papers*, edited by David Solomon, 171–82. Indianapolis: Bobbs-Merrill, 1966.

Stanford, Derek. "Introduction." In *Hashish, Wine, Opium: Théophile Gautier and Charles Baudelaire*, v–xx. London: One World Classics, 2009.

Steindl-Rast, David. "Psychoactive Substances and Sacred Values: Reconsidering Abraham Maslow's Discoveries." In *Seeking the Sacred with Psychoactive Substances: Chemical Paths to Spirituality and to God*, edited by J. Harold Ellens, 381–94. Santa Barbara, CA: Praeger, 2014.

Stern, Madeleine. "Introduction." In *Louisa May Alcott Unmasked: Collected Thrillers*, edited by Madeleine Stern, xi–xxix. Boston: Northeastern University Press, 1995.

Stux, Gabriel, Brian Berman, and Bruce Pomeranz. *Basics of Acupuncture*. Berlin: Springer, 2003.

Suzuki, Daisetsu Teitaro. *Selected Works of D. T. Suzuki, Volume I: Zen*. Berkeley: University of California Press, 2014.

Suzuki, Shunryu. *Zen Mind, Beginners Mind*. New York: Weatherhill, 1995.

Svoboda, Robert, and Arnie Lade. *Tao and Dharma: Chinese Medicine and Ayurveda*. Twin Lakes, WI: Lotus Press, 1995.

Tignor, Robert. *Egypt: A Short History*. Princeton, NJ: Princeton University Press, 2010.

Tolkien, J. R. R. *Unfinished Tales of Númenor and Middle-Earth*. New York: Ballantine, 1980.

Tolle, Eckhart. *The Power of Now*. Vancouver: Namaste, 2004.

Touw, Mia. "The Religious and Medical Uses of Cannabis in China, India, and Tibet." *Journal of Psychoactive Drugs* 13.1 (1981): 23–34.

Urbina, Ian. "Blacks Are Singled Out for Marijuana Arrests, Federal Data Suggests." *New York Times*, June 3, 2013. http://www.nytimes.com/2013/06/04/us/marijuana-arrests-four-times-as-likely-for-blacks.html.

Waley, Arthur, trans. *The Book of Songs*. New York: Grove, 1996.

Wallace, Vesna A. *The Inner Kālacakratantra: A Buddhist Tantric View of the Individual*. Oxford: Oxford University Press, 2001.

Walsh, Roger. "The Religious Use of Psychedelic Experiences in Shamanism and the Question of the Value and Validity of Such Experiences." In *Seeking the Sacred with Psychoactive Substances: Chemical Paths to Spirituality and to God*, edited by J. Harold Ellens, 169–78. Santa Barbara, CA: Praeger, 2014.

Watts, Alan. *The Art of Contemplation*. New York: Pantheon, 1972.

———. *The Joyous Cosmology: Adventures in the Chemistry of Consciousness*. New York: New World, 2013.

Watts, David. *The Psychedelic Experience: A Sociological Study*. Beverly Hills: Sage, 1971.

Weil, Andrew. *The Natural Mind: A New Way to Look at Drugs and the Higher Consciousness*. New York: Houghton Mifflin, 1972.

Williams-Garcia, Roberto. "The Ritual Use of Cannabis in Mexico." In *Cannabis and Culture*, edited by Vera Rubin, 133–45. Paris: Mouton, 1975.

Wilson, Peter Lamborn. *Scandal: Essays in Islamic Heresy*. Brooklyn, NY: Autonomedia, 1988.

Winkelman, Michael. "Evolutionary Views of Entheogenic Consciousness." In *Seeking the Sacred with Psychoactive Substances: Chemical Paths to Spirituality and to God*, edited by J. Harold Ellens, 341–64. Santa Barbara, CA: Praeger, 2014.

———. "Shamanistic Consciousness and Human Evolution." In *Seeking the Sacred with Psychoactive Substances: Chemical Paths to Spirituality and to God*, edited by J. Harold Ellens, 129–55. Santa Barbara, CA: Praeger, 2014.

Wonderley, Anthony. *Oneida Iroquois Folklore, Myth, and History: New York Oral Narrative from the Notes of H. E. Allen and Others*. Syracuse, NY: Syracuse University Press, 2004.

Yaden, David, and Andrew Newberg. "A New Means for Perennial Ends: Self-Transcendent Experiences and Noninvasive Brain Stimulation." In *Seeking the Sacred with Psychoactive Substances: Chemical Paths to Spirituality and to God*, edited by J. Harold Ellens, 303–24. Santa Barbara, CA: Praeger, 2014.

Yang, Shou-zhong. *The Divine Farmer's Materia Medica: A Translation of the Shen Nong Ben Cao Jing*. Boulder, CO: Blue Poppy Press, 2007.

Yazaki, Saeko. *Islamic Mysticism and Abū Ṭālib Al-Makkī: The Role of the Heart*. New York: Routledge, 2013.

Yeats, W. B. *Autobiography: Consisting of Reveries over Childhood and Youth, The Trembling of the Veil, and Dramatis Personae*. New York: Macmillan, 1953.

Zaehner, R. C. *Hindu Scriptures*. London: Everyman, 1966.

INDEX

Afghanistan, 12, 32, 45
Agni, 16, 17
Ahura Mazdā, 33, 33–34, 35
Al-Bisṭāmī, 40–41
Al-Ghazālī, 42–44
Al-Ḥallāj, 41
Al-Is'irdī, 47–48
Al-Sulami, 41–42
Alan Watts, 6, 43–44, 106, 135, 136
alchemy, 62–63, 65, 66, 135
alcohol, 7, 28, 29, 40, 56, 96, 125, 143, 152–153
Alcott, Louise May, 132, 134, 147
Alpert, Richard (Ram Dass), 6
animism, 6, 12, 17, 20, 66
asceticism, 27, 39
Ashoka, 12, 13
Ātman, 20–21, 22–23, 25, 95
Avesta (or *Zend-Avesta*), 7, 32–33, 34–35
Ayurvedic medicine, 29, 55, 56, 66, 68, 99

Babylon, 92–93, 95, 96, 97
Bantu peoples, 78, 80, 84
Baudelaire, Charles, 8, 126, 127–129, 134, 135; *Artificial Paradises* (*Les paradis artificiels*), 128, 138
Bena-Riamba, 7, 84–85
Benjamin, Walter, 134, 137–139
Bhagavad Gītā, 15, 23–24, 28, 64, 99; Arjuna in, 23–26
Blake, William, 36, 136, 139, 155

Book of Songs (*Shijing*), 7, 51–54, 99
Böhme, Jakob, 136, 154
Bön, 66, 99
botanicals, 17, 66, 73, 110, 117, 152
Bowles, Paul, 143
Brahmā, 20
Brahman, 19–21, 22–23, 25, 28, 64, 95
Brāhman priests, 17, 19, 27
Buddhism, 141; Indian, 12, 27, 55, 56; Tibetan, 7, 66–68, 99; Zen, 5, 42, 48, 103

Cao Cao, 56
Caribbean, 29, 89, 92, 96, 97, 99
caste, 11, 16, 17, 24, 26, 27
China, 7, 12, 48, 51, 55, 56, 66, 69, 98. *See also* Traditional Chinese Medicine
Christianity, 1–8, 35, 36, 87, 88, 106, 120, 135, 136; doctrines, 34, 119, 123, 129; Gnostic, 74–76; history of, 37, 73, 76–77, 88, 96, 108; in New World, 115–116; monastic tradition, 39, 87, 99, 122
Christopher Columbus, 89
coffee, 126, 152
colonialism, 13; in Africa, 77, 80, 82, 87, 89; in the Americas, 89, 91, 92, 115
Colorado, 1, 3, 149
Confucius (Kongzi), 52
Congo, 83, 84, 88
Constantine, 76